Dr. Sebi Natural Guide

The Essential Diet to Prevent Diseases and Stay Healthy With Fasting Plans and Herbal Treatments

Caroline Rollins

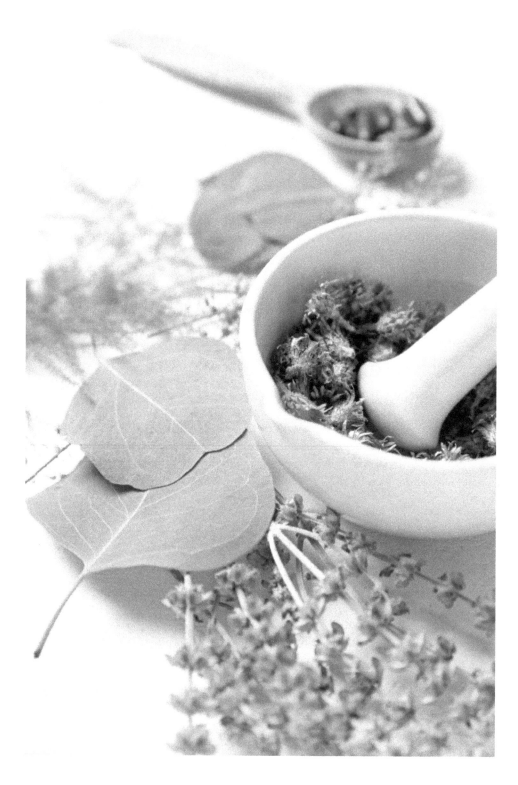

processes, or directions contained within is the solitary and utter responsibility of the recipient reader. Under no circumstances will any legal responsibility or blame be held against the publisher for reparation, damages, or monetary loss due to the information herein, either directly or indirectly.

Respective authors own all copyrights not held by the publisher.

The information herein is offered for informational purposes solely and is universal as such. The presentation of the information is without a contract or any guarantee assurance.

The trademarks used are without any consent, and the publication of the trademark is without permission or backing by the trademark owner. All trademarks and brands within this book are for clarifying purposes only and are owned by the owners themselves, not affiliated with this document.

Contents

Dr. Sebi Fasting

A Guide To Dr.Sebi Diet And Fasting For Healing And Detoxification Of Your Body.

Introduction

Study findings have demonstrated that our health can be improved by a diet focused on plants. In a study in 2015, a vegan diet resulted in greater weight loss than other diets that were less stringent. The participants lost up to 7.5 percent of their body weight after six months on a vegan diet. Concerning appetite control, a 2016 survey of young males

Participants agreed that they felt fuller and more satisfied than a meat meal after eating a meal of plants containing peas and beans. A plant-based diet could favorably modify the microbiome in a 2019 study, leading to reduced disease risk. A 2017 research also found that herbal diets could decrease the risk of coronary heart disease by 40 percent and the risk of developing metabolic syndrome and type 2 diabetes by half. The diet of Dr. Sebi encourages individuals to eat whole foods and prevents food production. Research in 2017 showed that reducing refined food intake in the United States would improve the nutritional consistency of the general diet. The diet of Dr. Sebi does not contain adequate essential nutrients that the diet website does not mention. They can benefit from seeing a healthcare provider who may recommend more supplements if they eat this diet. Following Dr. Sebi's diet, vitamin B-12 deficiency may result. Through eating vitamins and fortified foods, an individual can prevent this. Vitamin B-12 is an important nutrient required for the health of nerves and blood cells, and DNA development. In general, people who adopt vegetarian diets and older adults are presented with the possibility of B-12 deficiency. For those who do not eat meat products, doctors usually recommend B-12 supplements. In the hands and feet, B-12 deficiency symptoms include fatigue, depression, and tingling.

There is also a risk of pernicious anemia that prevents enough red blood cells from being formed by the body. Nutrition contributes to the brain's well-being, in the diet, muscles, bones, hormones, and DNA. In line with current directives, 46 g of protein consumption is expected for women over 19 years of age, while 56 g is expected for men of the same age. Protein in all of Dr. Sebi's diet items. One hundred grams of oven-red chicken breast contains, for comparison, 16.79 g of nutrients. Dr. Sebi's diet, however, limits other types of plant proteins, such as peanuts, lenses, and soy. To meet everyday needs, a person would have to eat an exceedingly significant amount of the permitted protein sources.

Research indicates that to ingest adequate amino acids that constitute protein blocks, it is necessary to eat various plant foods. For cell membrane materials, Omega-3 fatty acids are also important. The diet for Dr. Sebi requires sources of omega-3 plants, such as hemp and walnuts. A replacement of omega-3 will help anyone who practices Dr. Sebi's diet. Dr. Sebi's preparations often contain botanical herbs that are rare or patented. However, a person who does not strictly adhere to the diet can easily adapt such recipes to produce healthy, herbal food. Remember to leave out the date sugar for Dr. Sebi's 'veggie-fuel' smoothie, as the drink can be sweet enough without it. Maple syrup or chocolate sugar can be used to replace the sugar dates. Tortillas may be favored by those who consume wheat or maize. Scientific experiments do not validate the diet of Dr. Sebi. It does, however, deliver some of the benefits of other diets focused on vegetables. There may be positive health benefits from further consumption of whole fruits and vegetables. If that's a goal, it can also make a person lose weight. The limits on

Dr. Sebi's diet, however, could pose dangers. It is important to ensure that sufficient nutrients, including vitamin B-12, are provided to the body if necessary. Any people may be more vulnerable to the risks of Dr. Sebi's diet. Kids, mothers who breastfeed, and older adults are among them.

Diet proponents recommend lavish goods that are not supported by scientific evidence. A safer option could be more vegetable-based diets and any absent nutrients. For a healthcare provider, researching and consulting before trying a new diet may be smart practice. This GUIDE discusses the makeup and effects of following Dr. Sebi's diet into a gradual detoxification process to revitalize the body. Let's start.

Chapter 1: Introduction to Dr. Sebi and Dr. Sebi Diet

Identified as Dr. Sebi, Alfredo Bowman was a self-proclaimed Honduran herbalist. He was self-educated and, according to his website, had no formal physician qualifications. He hadn't been a surgeon,

He didn't hold a doctorate either. He emigrated to the United States and was unsuccessfully treated for numerous health conditions, including diabetes, asthma, impotence, and obesity. His website claims that he was healed in Mexico by a herbalist who influenced him to create his herbal blends, called Cell Food by Dr. Sebi. He initially believed his herbs would cure autoimmune diseases such as AIDS, sickle cell anemia, and lupus, according to the Health Line. But in 1987, he was accused of practicing medicine without a license (although the jury acquitted him). After another allegation by

A few years back, in New York, Sebi agreed to avoid saying that all diseases could be healed by his medicines. Sebi's client list allegedly included, albeit controversial: John Travolta, Michael Jackson, and Steven Seagal. Sebi was apprehended for money laundering in 2016. He contracted pneumonia during his detention in Honduras and died on his way to the hospital. The man who worked on his documentary, Nipsey Hussle, was also killed, while others took his death and Sebi's as evidence of the plotting of shadow forces to undermine the reality of Sebi's remedies. The main conviction of Sebi assumes that alkaline foods and herbs (pH> 7) are essential to balance the acid in our bodies, so maintaining this alkaline condition prevents us from the buildup of mucus that contributes to illness. The alkaline coronation, like our long-awaited Savior, shows a deep misunderstanding of the human body.

1.1. Sebi-African bio-minerals

Simply placed, Sebi's Cell Food products are herbs, fungi, and algae branded as African Bio-Mineral Balance products; a bottle of Bromide Plus capsules containing "Irish sea moss" and the bladderwrack is available for $30. All of these ingredients may be linked to allergies, intolerance, or prescription. I don't know the big burden. Many Sebi compounds are sold as a detoxification solution, but we should know our body doesn't require regular detoxification. We are advised the toxins are already vague and not well-defined, but we never saw the detox methods we offer impact these disgusting boogeymen. "The gene resonates electrically in Africa." Sadly, Sebi's wellbeing belief went beyond traditional nonsense and race pseudoscience. Sebi also stated that African genes have high resonance and naturally "compliments [sic] the African gene structure." Genes are non-resonant. You can ask about your genetic ancestry packs, telling you that your parents originated from Ireland and Tunisia. While their accuracy is at stake, they look for single-letter changes around the genome and compare the trend with a reference population representing itself in one area. Pure driving is the idea of genes vibrating at such

frequencies that determine the dietary needs. The internet is full of self-trained gurus who profess to be every disease's sole true cause and panacea. Unfortunately, real science steadily traces, drawing the image of a complicated universe in which various illnesses have different origins, and treatments are flawed, sometimes causing side effects.

1.2. What is the Dr. Sebi Diet?

Sebi believed diseases are caused by mucus and body acidity and argued that diseases could not be found in an alkaline climate. This plan, which involves a strict diet and pricey supplements, claims to restore alkalinity AND detoxify the body. The diet restricts animal products and concentrates on vegan food, but with much tighter laws. It limits seedless berries, for instance, and only allows Sebi's approved list of "natural growing grains." Here's a shortlist of his diet guide's foods: Vegetables: Amaranth greens, chayotes, avocado, cucumber, garbanzo beans, isots, dandelions greens, kale, lettuce (all but Iceberg), nopales, okra, olives, onions, mushrooms (all except shiitake), sea vegetables, squash, tomatoes. Fruit: Apples, bananas, berries (all kinds of fruits), cantaloupes, elderberries cereals, currants, dates, figs, grapes of grapes, lime, oranges, peaches, pears, mangoes, melons feathers, pears, plums, soft gelatos, soursops (seeds), tamarind pears, raisins, soft gourd cocoa Herbal teas: burdock, fennel, ginger, chamomile, fennel, raspberry, linden. Plants: Amaranth, quinoa, rye, fonio, Kamut. Nuts, seeds: raw sesame seeds, hemp seeds, raw sonic butter, "tahini" walnuts, Brazilian nuts.

Oils: Olive oil (not cook pasta oil, sesame oil), coconut oil, hemp oil, avocado oil. Basil, garlic, dill, orange, savory, leavened bread, sweet basil, achiote, cayenne, tarragon, thyme, onion powder, pure sea salt, habanero, sage, pure agave syrup, sugar date.

Sebi's diet guide also contains several other rules: You can only eat food listed in Sebi's Nutrition Guide. One gallon of natural spring water must be drunk every day. All animal products, including dairy, fish, and "hybrid" foods, are forbidden. Alcohol is not allowed. Sebi foods must be taken one hour before drugs. You must avoid wheat and consume only the "natural-growing grains" No fruit (canned or seedless) is permitted. Microwaves should be stopped.

Is Dr. Sebi Diet sound?

The diet is extremely protein deficient: Sebi does not tolerate animals' fats, eggs, milk, or even soy. It also restricts the bulk of legumes and beans. The only protein in the diet is some hemp seeds, walnuts, "natural growing grains," and brazil nuts. Satisfying the nutritional requirements of these items alone can be very difficult. Protein is an integral part of all the cells in your body, and for tissue building and healing, the body needs protein. An essential part of muscles, bones, flesh, blood, and cartilage is protein. It may lead to malnutrition by limiting macronutrients and major food groups.

Although it supports certain fruits and vegetables, several things are strangely diminished. Cherry or plum tomatoes are permitted, for instance, but there are no other kinds. Some kinds of products include lettuce and shiitake mushrooms, making it much more difficult to adopt the diet. The primary emphasis of Sebi is on his supplements that pledge "revitalize and engage intercellular advancement and "expedite the healing process. Some packets cost up to $1,500, and nutrient and quantity details are not specified. Which makes it impossible to know how much you get from its patented mixtures and exactly what is in its supplements. In any way, Sebi is not a doctor, and there is no evidence-based research available to support his claims and guidelines. His extremely stringent dietary recommendations promote the eradication of certain foods.

The diet also recommends taking supplements to Dr. Sebi Cell Food. Dietary rules:

1. If the food is not in the "Nutritional Guide." it is not recommended.
2. All Dr. Sebi's things can be taken together without a trace.
3. The best results for a disease reversal are strict adherence to the' Dietary Guide' (with supplementary products).
4. Agricultural products, hybrid crops, dried fruit, seedless fruits, or beer are not eaten.
5. According to Sebi, you use the microwave to "kill your food" avoid it.

What does body alkalization mean?

The principle of balancing the pH of your body through the food you consume is an alkaline diet. The belief is that waste can have a pH ranging between acidic and alkaline when used in our bodies. The human body has varying pH ratios in different regions, with organs such as the most acidic stomach and more alkaline blood. Urines are a blood pH-management mediated body product directly affected by the food we eat. The larger "alkaline diets" group focuses on the metabolic waste problem, and the diets of Dr. Sebi are among many and safe for consuming nutritious plant foods. Still, there is little truth behind the body's alkalization, and his argument is not confirmed by science. Although the diet makes substantial claims, it cannot be proven. As an alternative diet based on vegetables, it can lead to comparable advantages where the benefits are best explored, but protein sources prefer not to have a strict dietary schedule. If you are contemplating trying a diet based on vegetables, you can anticipate several benefits. Here are few ideas to get your journey underway. Here's a full list of Dr. Sebi's diet foods if you are interested:

Plants

- Amaranth Greens
- Chayote (a Mexican squash)
- Kürbis
- Greens Dandelion
- Garbanzo beans
- Izote (cactus flowers/leaves)
- Mushrooms (but not shiitake)
- Nopales
- Okra
- Olives
- Onions

- Wonderful seafood
- Squash
- The peppers (only cherry or plum varieties)
- Tomatillos
- Toxins in zucchini
- Buggy Baby (verdolaga)

Fruit

- Apples
- Banana
- Beers
- Cantaloupe
- Cherries
- Dates
- Varieties of grapes
- Limes
- Mango
- Melons
- Orange
- Papayas
- Pear pinching
- Prunes
- Young coconut.

Oils

- Olive oil
- Coconut oil
- grapefruit Oil
- Sesame Oil
- Hempseed Oil

Noodles and seeds

- Hemp seeds
- Crude sesame seeds
- Raw Tahini
- Brazilian Nuts

Seasoning

- Basilique
- Bay Leaf
- Dill
- Savory
- Sweet Basil
- Tarragon
- Thyme
- Cayenne
- powdered Onion

- The Havanese
- Pure sea salt
- Pure agave syrup
- Saccharose Date

Teas

- The Kurds
- Chamomile
- Elderberry
- Fennel
- Raspberry

Chapter 2: Acidity of Human Body and Alkaline and Acid Balance through Dr. Sebi Diet

In schools across the USA, educators use litmus paper tests to show that pH ranges between acidity and alkalinity. Is the concept of acidity and alkalinity, therefore, applicable to real life? Yeah, since there is a survival pH for any aspect of the human body. Individuals must also encourage the correct pH in their bodies. In various mineral solutions with a pH scale of 0 to 14, scientists have developed acidity or alkalinity measurements. Every acidic solution with a pH lower than 7.0 is acidic with the highest acidity pH. Any solution having a pH greater than 7.0 is alkaline, with an alkaline pH of 14. The human body retains a mildly alkaline state when it is healthy. The pH in our blood is 7.4. If the blood pH decreases to 7.0, he or she is killed by major organ failure. A steady blood pH of 7.4 is needed by organs like the heart, lungs, and brain. Therefore, when any cell in the human body resides, respires, and waste exists, the human body constantly works to preserve the correct pH, and these waste products are usually acidic. In certain cases, if the body absorbs too much acidic food, if the cells contain too much acidic waste, or if these acids may not be removed or neutralized by the body, the body can become too dangerously acidic. The cells bathe in their waste if the acids cannot be neutralized or expelled. This disorder is referred to as acidosis or excess acidity. In the heart membranes, nerve and vein cells, acidosis erodes and consumes in such a manner that acid steadily moves through some of the world's hardest materials, such as marble or metal. The slow erosion and decay of the body's cells are responsible for many cancers and premature aging.

2.1. Acidity and the Pancreas

Naturally, somebody's parts are more alkaline than others. The most susceptible to acidic exposure are highly alkaline glands, such as the Liver and Pancreas. There is a pH of 7.8 to 8.0 in the pancreatic juice. The pH of the liver bile is from 7.5 to 8.8. But both pancreatic and bile juices get more acidic as the body's acidity increases. Bile and acidic pancreatic juices, stones, ulcers, and pancreatic and liver tissue cancer are the destructive, irritating, and inflammatory causes of acidosis. The reflux or bile backflow into the Pancreas, bladder, throat, and esophagus is often caused by excessively acidic bile. The duodenum and stomach are also linked with bile reflux, leading to diarrhea, ulcers, and cancer. Often, acid reflux and bile reflux arise simultaneously, inflaming the esophagus and increasing esophageal cancer risk. Bile pancreas reflux is another problem for elevated total acid toxicity, or where the bile is in the Pancreas. This bile backup will cause acute pancreatitis and make problems with chronic pancreatitis worse. In gallbladder stone processing, acidic bile is also considered an important element. It can cause severe pancreatic damage and hepatic damage by blocking the pancreas and bile ducts. Minerals and bicarbonates are impossible for pancreatic cells to receive as blood becomes too acidic to make adequate alkaline pancreatic juice. There are some issues without alkaline pancreatic juice: fewer pancreatic enzymes induce duodenum indigestion and decreased activity of the protease inhibitor (the special enzymes that suppress protease from the digestion of its Pancreas within the own pancreatic duct). Inflammation of pancreatitis starts as the protease digests the pancreatic cells, increases Pancreas of calcium that helps irritate pancreas stones, and reduces anti-microbial properties of pancreatic juice spasm and the resultant blockage of Oddi sphincter. This blockage increases the pancreatic pressure, which, through trapped digestive enzymes, begins the digestion of pancreatic cells. This causes pain, inflammation which may result in the death of the Pancreas.

Good pancreas food, minerals: Normally, our present diet is acidic and shifts the body's pH balance to an acidic state known as metabolic acidosis. When natural alkaline diets, such as fresh vegetables, migrate away from the usual US diet, metabolic acidosis becomes more common. The body becomes acidic with acid-producing foods such as beef, certain dairy products, white meals, sugar, tobacco, processed vegetable oils, soft drinks, and coffee. Acidity is also caused by stress, sedentary living conditions, smoking, free radicals, systemic inflammation and infection. With an elevated over-acidity level, the disorder is considered a dangerous disease that weakens the whole body. To neutralize and dispose of high acidity, the body must absorb alkaline minerals from key tissues, bones, and muscles. These minerals, including calcium, magnesium, sodium, and potassium, have positive health characteristics. The Pancreas is annoyed, inducing infection and cancer when the Pancreas spills these essential minerals and bicarbonates. To reduce over-acidity of the body, more minerals and bicarbonates have to be incorporated into the diet. Via the treatment of food and mineral water, these minerals and bicarbonates are extracted.

The way we eat today is entirely distinct from the diet and dietary habits of our ancestors. All facets of our lives, including what we eat, have altered technology and its growth. In the busy world that we work in, fast food is the norm. The lifestyle embraced by our ancestors is entirely the reverse of carrying out meals, preparing easily with the processed food we buy in our supermarkets, and dietary habits, such as eating while watching TV. The result is that fewer fruits and vegetables are eaten, and more refined products, milk products and protein from animal meat are consumed simultaneously. With crash diets and low starch diets of high protein, we compensate with what we eat. Then we ask why ailments like cardiac disorders, different allergies, and bone diseases, which were not so prevalent years ago, have become a reality in our lives. Doctors, nutritionists, and dieticians think the body is influenced by what you consume and can be associated with specific diseases, such as those mentioned above. Food affects our bodies' metabolism and how it functions each day. False foods can damage the body, creating issues with health due to body imbalance. Thus, these health issues can be reversed or preferably prevented by modifying our practices on what we eat.

2.2. Alkaline and Acid Balance

All foods affect the levels of acid/alkaline in the body. Acids must be balanced for good health to be maintained. For strength, endurance, and energy, the body should be slightly alkaline. Natural health is revitalized and promoted by an alkaline diet. The term pH is "Potential of Hydrogen," which calculates the relative acidity or alkalinity. The pH level indicates the acid/alkaline balance of the body and informs the individual's health. The scale for pH runs from 0-14. Zero is entirely acidic, and 14 are alkaline. The middle scale, 7, is neutral. High-quality water has a pH of 7. An individual is very rarely too alkaline. In someone who eats little to no protein, it's more common. The issue is more acidic, however, for the vast majority. Slightly alkaline blood should be (7.34- 7.45). This range means disease and is acidic below 7.0 pH. The pH above 7.0 is alkaline. Because of consuming too many proteins and carbohydrates, one must be careful not to build an acidic pH equilibrium. An acidic pH can induce too much discomfort. Too many toxins from the body that take oxygen and nutrients from cells can also produce an acidic equilibrium.

Acidic consequences of equilibrium:

- The ability of the body to absorb minerals and nutrients is weakened.
- Heightened radical damage.
- Mental clarity declines.
- Physical energy is diminishing.
- It is normal to have insomnia and disrupted sleep patterns.
- Impairment of the immune system as assistive intestinal bacteria die.
- There are common colds, illnesses, and influenza.
- Usually, most strawberries, green vegetables, carrots, beans, lentils, spices, seasonings, berries, and nuts are alkaline foods.

- Beef, fish, poultry, chickens, and legumes are acid-forming foods.
- Drink eight-10 glasses of water daily.

Meditation, tai chi, reflexology, massage, acupuncture, soothing touch, relaxing music, and yoga are activities that buffer daily acids and support an alkaline body. Your mental state is also a vital health factor and can affect your pH.

2.3. Dr. Sebi Diet and PH balance

Dr. Sebi recommends Alkaline Diet. Alkaline diet strategy includes the development as follows:

A. 75% alkaline foods with a pH above 7.4, as close to eight; and

B. 25% acidic foods.

What's the difference between acidic and alkaline foods?

The internal pH (blood) usually is 7.38-7, 52. The pH does not decrease. Below 7, since grade IV coma and patient death may be caused by this. The blood also doesn't have to have a very basic but just marginally alkaline character. Otherwise, the risk of spontaneous muscle contractions is exceedingly intense and painful.

What foods are alkaline, acidic?

In the alkaline diet group, we have:

A. Cheese, avocado cucumbers and lettuce, and all chlorophyll-rich vegetables;

B. Soy milk, lemon, millet, coconut, beans, and buckwheat;

C. Sea buckthorn's; and

D. Some cold-pressed oil;

Alkaline water is key to diet!

It is advised that those who are unable to meet the prescribed nutritional ratio (25 percent acidic and 75 percent alkaline foods) should be asked to eat alkaline water replacement drinks.

Any water with a pH greater than 7.7 is known to be alkaline water and can be consumed significantly. There is a very low chance of raising the blood's pH to critical values; 2.5-3 liters of alkaline water a day can help maintain good wellbeing and help detoxify the body and clear free radicals.

Smoking is forbidden!

Smoking is a habit that boosts the acidity of the liver, which happens when we drink alcohol. These habits are often advised to be minimized or removed from daily life so that the body can remain healthy and clean. On alkaline diets, smoking is strictly banned.

Did you know the traditional Western diet consists of acid? This suggests that our diets cause a phenomenal blood deficiency, and did you know it could be incredibly detrimental to your health? The body is made up of 70 percent liquids, as you may know. Hydrogen potential(pH) is a calculation of solution acidity or alkalinity. The higher the pH, the wealthiest fluid is more alkaline and oxygen.

The lower the pH, the fluid is less acidic and oxygen. When our diets are high in acid-forming ingredients, however, our diets lack ample alkaline content to compensate, the acid starts to build up in our cells, allowing them to be depleted of oxygen and die. Suppose our body does not have the perfect pH, so vitamins and minerals cannot successfully heal or assimilate themselves. PH levels influence all, so the alkaline pH equilibrium has to be retained much of the time.

Hold your urine in pH bands that you can shop online or in health food shops and measure your pH levels. To ensure that your pH level is correctly expressed, we urge you to monitor your levels more than once a day and monitor your readings for several weeks. If your pH levels dip below 7.0 much of the day, the consumption of nutritious green vegetables, salads, sprouts, and fruit needs to be improved. Raw food is better because it is filled with vitamins, minerals, and enzymes that kill the heat.

Acidic pH levels, some of which are listed below, can cause many

health problems:

- Weight gain, obesity, and diabetes
- Immune deficiency
- Hormonal problems
- Slow digestion and treatment
- Bad hair, skin, clots
- Lack of energy and fatigue
- There are dying muscles, cramps, and spasms.

- Allergies, infections, and ulcers
- Depressing trends

The list goes on.

The list of health complaints may seem far too familiar, but it is important to know, and relatively easily, that the ideal pH level can be achieved. Cut down on dairy, meat, pasta, bread, rice, tea, coffee, and alcohol (all acidic foods) and increase your consumption of fresh raw fruit and vegetables (alkalizing foods).

Try dietary supplements of 60 percent alkaline food, up to 40 percent (maximum) acidic foods. We recommend many raw fruits and vegetables as snacks, as they are alkaline and help you lose weight, regain energy, and are healthy and delicious!

Chapter 3: Dr. Sebi Fasting following Alkaline Diet

You will consume lots of food during the Dr. Sebi or Alkaline Fasting! This form of medication for detox or cleaning is not about consuming as little or just drinking water as possible, but about eating the right stuff. Usually, a diet schedule requires multiple meals a day, mostly of organic foods, balanced plants, berries high in minerals, seeds or nuts. On the dish, nearly anything that is raw, vegetable, and unprocessed, without additives, is permitted. Therefore, eating alkaline food for a while is by no means one-sided - but more diverse and colorful!

3.1. Forbidden foods on Dr. Sebi Fasting

You'll have to skip certain food items used in traditional meals and recipes when preparing your alkaline diet menu. It is specifically illegal to use all foods that contain acidity in the body. Misleadingly, foods exempt from the alkaline diet, such as lemons containing acid, are not sour tasting but rather processed sugar or dairy products.

- Meat
- Fish

- Milk products

- Grain products (white flour products)

- Legumes

- Sugar

- Coffee

- Alcohol

3.2. Is it Dr. Sebi Fasting or Intermittent Fasting Following Dr. Sebi Diet?

The fasting pattern followed in Dr. Sebi Fasting is similar to that of Intermittent Fasting patterns. It's just that you have to follow Dr. Sebi Diet and meal plans during intermittent fasting eating cycles.

3.3. Forms of Fasting and Intermittent Fasting

Since the 1930s, we've learned that by limiting what a mouse eats, you can extend its life, but it wasn't until recently that we could be sure that it would work with an animal that was more like us. Scientists released the findings of a completely long-term study on the mouse lemur in June 2018. Notwithstanding the name, mouse lemurs have little to do with rodents. They are apes, which means that monkeys and humans are members of the same extended family. They are relatively short-lived (which is convenient if you are researching aging) and are close to ours in their body chemistry. Many mouse lemurs were taken and split into two classes by researchers from the National Institute of Aging to do their experiment. In common scenarios and on the same nutritious diets, the classes were brought up. The only distinction was that one group was made to survive 30 percent fewer calories than the other group from early adulthood (the control group). What happened, then? Yeah, the gaps became more and more apparent as the years passed on. Young-looking and glossy, the calorie-restricted lemurs persisted. They had significantly lower cancer and diabetes rates, and checks on their mental skills indicated that they kept on the ball. Brain scans have shown that a lot more white matter, the synaptic fibers linking various brain regions, had been retained than the lemurs on a normal diet. Most remarkable of all, they lived 50 years longer on average than their cousins, who were better fed. This is fairly compelling proof that the limitation of calories will prolong an animal's life like humans. When the last animal in the test community died, about a third of the calorie-controlled animals were still alive.

3.4. More Manageable Forms of Fasting

It may prolong your life, but it is not something most of us aim to pursue after a Calorie Restriction Optimum Nutrition lifestyle. People following this lifestyle are called **CRONies.** Without the negatives, I like the perks of calorie restriction. And that's why intermittent fasting is so exciting for us. It appears to deliver all of the advantages of long-term calorie restriction by cutting your calories for brief amounts of time or limiting when you eat your calories. And it's a lot simpler and much more convenient than that.

We are going to update you with the latest science in this section of the book.

Three of the most common ways of intermittent fasting are as follows:

Periodic fasting (where, once every few months, you cut your food down

for five days in a row).

The 5:2 approach (Restricting calories for two days a week).

Time-Restricted Eating (Restricting your eating to a narrow time window).

Different health advantages are offered for both of these types of intermittent fasting.

And what's better is that they aren't mutually exclusive. Let's look at every single one of them.

3.5. Periodic Fasting

Professor Valter Longo, head of the Longevity Center of the University of Southern California, is one of the world's foremost authorities on the study of human aging. He was also one of the first scientists I went to look for answers to what fasting is, how it operates, and why it is important for human health. Large, lean and aged well, Valter is perfect advertising for his study. He was born in 1967 in Italy and looked ten years younger than his actual age. Valter believes passionately in using fasting's ability to slow aging and discourage infectious illnesses such as cancer, heart disease, and diabetes from arising. He has devoted his life to studying the processes by which this arises. And the positive thing is that he believes that we now have a pretty good idea of when and how to postpone aging. Best still, to live a long and healthy life, you don't have to give up eating well or become a skinny CRONie. Then why is fasting one of the most powerful things you can do, as Valter said to me once?

Autophagy

The list of things fasting does to your body is long and nuanced, but one of the most striking advantages is that it stimulates a mechanism called 'autophagy' within the body, which simply means 'self-eat.' Autophagy is a fully normal mechanism in which cells that are dead, diseased or worn-out are broken down and engulfed. Think of the body as a little bit like a vehicle. It's bright and sparkling because it's new and it all works. Yet pieces get worn out as time goes by, and certain parts tend to rust. If you insist on constantly pushing it around at high speed, so it will finally fall apart. You need to take it to a dealership so that technicians can repair and install worn-out pieces and spruce it up to keep the vehicle running for as long as possible. The simple fact is that, at the same time, you can't fix your vehicle and run it hard. The same happens to us. Much like we need sleep, if we want to toggle on the repair genes that keep us in good health, we need time off from constant feeding. It is only because we do not consume or drink food with calories that our bodies can continue this repair process. Autophagy is caused by fasting, and as time goes by, it gets more severe. When you eat, it ends.

Regeneration

Autophagy is stimulated by fasting, which means the body will clear the junk and garbage, i.e., old cells, out. But when you start to eat, what happens? Is all the good that you did, then, undone? Valter and his friends experimented to find out in 2014. 8 For two days at a time, over several months, they took a group of mice and made them fast. One of the first things that happened was that they began dropping their white blood cell count. This was an anticipated and safe reaction, as Valter explained. Your system wants to conserve energy while you fast, and one of the things it does is recycle a lot of the immune cells that are not required, especially those that are old or weakened.' So what happened when after their fast, the mice were able to feed? With the formation of new, more active white cells, their bodies quickly responded. 'We couldn't have expected,' Valter said, 'that fasting will have such a remarkable effect.' It seems that fasting often provides room for new cells to develop by causing Autophagy. It's like a forest fire that burns the old undergrowth down, making room for new trees and plants.

Fasting, accompanied by feeding, gives the body the 'okay' to go on and start producing fresh cells. Therefore, if the immune system is not as strong as it once was (either because you are elderly or because you have undergone medical care, such as chemotherapy), it can be regenerated by brief periods of fasting.

3.6. The 5:2 Approach

Periodic fasting may be a perfect way to restart the immune system, and for patients undergoing chemotherapy, it could turn out to be very beneficial, but we were searching for something different: a simple way to lose weight and reverse diabetes. So back in 2012, we came up with our method of intermittent fasting after talking to tons of other scientists, which we felt would be healthier and more doable. We used to call it the '5:2 diet.' We determined that we would eat healthier for five days a week, and we would cut down to around 25 percent of our usual diet on our two fasting days, which would mean that we would eat about 600 calories a day. We didn't feel that the days we fasted would make any difference, so we opted for Tuesdays and Thursdays. This was primarily an elimination process. For apparent social motives, we didn't want to go on Fridays or weekends. Also, fasting on a Monday struck us as an unattractive way to begin the week. We wanted to do our back-to-back fasts (Tuesdays and Wednesdays), but we find it uncomfortable. Despite the somewhat haphazard way we came up with the 5:2 regime, we were shocked and pleased at how common and successful it has proven to be, not just for us but also for many other individuals. Such citizens as Natalia.

Natalia, who is 53, knew she wanted to do something after discovering a couple of years earlier that she was going up the stairs, out of breath. She went to the psychiatrist and was advised she had diabetes on a borderline basis. She was particularly concerned about that since her mom has type 2 diabetes. 'I saw a book of yours and followed it to the text. In the first eight weeks, I lost 16kg, and since then, I've lost another 6kg. I'm no longer a borderline diabetic, so I'm still better than I have ever been. "Yesterday, I saw my doctor, and he said I was a model patient." She adopted other healthier habits as she began to lose weight. This is always what exists. You turn to a virtuous cycle where you feel so much happier that you want to make improvements to your life, from getting wrapped up in a vicious cycle of fear and comfort eating. As Natalia told us, 'I've changed my sleep. More energetic, I thought. I continued with mindfulness. I entered a party cycling. I was put into swimming by the walking community.' So what stopped her on track? 'Knowing that I have taken the weight off and realizing that unless I'm patient, it will go back on. One of those people who are tall and slim who can eat loads of pizza is my husband. I realize I'm incapable. I did agree that. It's to acknowledge, in your head, that it's so vital that you should live your life differently.' Were there tough moments? 'The Lots. One evening, I recall vividly, I was walking around the house searching for a box of chocolate leftover from Christmas. Luckily, it was well concealed, so I finally gave up and just read a novel. My husband and children are very encouraging. They can see what a huge difference it has brought to my wellbeing and my confidence.'

3.7. Time Restricted Eating

Time-Limited Feeding is the final method of intermittent fasting that I want to educate you about (TRE). Recently, particularly among millennials, bodybuilders and celebrities, it has become famous. By doing a sort of TRE called 16:8, the actor Hugh Jackman says his Wolverine physique was made possible. I enjoy talking to the person trimming my locks while I get my hair trimmed. They all seem to be doing TRE these days. The TRE rules are very simple: you strive to ingest much of your calories within a narrow time, such as 12 hours (also known as 12:12). You don't eat or drink anything that includes calories beyond that duration until you have agreed on your time window (perhaps 9 am to 9 pm). By making your evening meal a bit earlier and your breakfast a bit later, you will start doing TRE (12:12). That way, you easily extend your usual overnight (the time you sleep and not eat) by a couple of hours. You can switch to 14:10 or even, like Hugh Jackman, to 16:8, once you've gotten used to this (where you eat all your calories in an eight-hour window, such as between midday and 8 pm, and fast for 16 hours).

3.8. Dr. Sebi's Alkaline Foods to Eat During Eating Windows While Fasting

The pH spectrum can be 0-14, with the highest acidity being zero and the highest alkalinity being 14. Of the food that we consume, our blood contains both acid and alkaline traces. Therefore, the optimal pH for a stable person is about 7.35-7.45. Our cells, muscles, lungs, and eventually our system can be affected even by a small decline in this amount. In order to survive, our cells require nutrients and enzymes, and these essential nutrients are provided by the food we eat. Some foods have higher levels of acid, and other foods have higher levels of alkali. Naturally, acidic foods will leave acid traces that will be incorporated into our blood cells. Instead, alkaline-rich foods leave alkaline deposits in our bodies. There is a clear correlation between eating correctly and keeping a healthy pH. Nature has supplied us with an abundance of food. There is no restriction to only a few kinds of fruits and vegetables, so we don't have to be sluggish to consume the same thing every day. We don't have to take it to be fit and strong by sticking to only one sort of food. We must assess the levels of alkalinity and acidity of different foods and balance them with our diets. Anthony Robbins has a catalog of foods that are alkaline and acidic, so it should not be difficult to launch this new diet plan. Our consumption of acidic foods and liquids should be decreased understandably, especially if we have already reached the acidic limit. Note that in our system, high acid levels can cause serious illnesses to develop. Oh, we have to bear in mind what our bodies are fed on. Using your list of alkaline ingredients, you will begin making healthy eating choices not only for yourself but for your mates. The basic idea of the pH miracle diet is to maintain a balanced pH. The fact that the human body is slightly alkaline is suitable for you to eat alkalizing foods. The digestive system gets unbalanced when you eat a bit too much acidic food. In addition, it induces many symptoms, including weight gain, depressed immunity, nausea, and poor focus, all of which can lead to more serious health conditions. Acidic foods (that are to be avoided), foods that are alkalizing (which are to be emphasized are the variables that affect the pH miracle diet. Alkalizing foods help maintain your body's pH and are, as a result, good for your body. Many people don't understand what pH, alkali, and acid mean and how they are associated with nutrition and health. The properties of alkalinity and acidity are called 'basic.' The cells that compose these foods decide these conditions. Therefore, the transition from alkaline to acid cannot be achieved by external treatment. Foods are alkaline or acidic at their foundation or base. Chemically, alkaline and acidic compounds are opposites. If there is an interaction between an acid and a base, a salt occurs. In a chemist's laboratory, these interactions are clear and simple.

However, the interaction is more complicated in our bodies due to the size with which the bases and acids meet. In either case, scientists have made several generalizations about the effects of alkaline compounds and acids in our digestive system. In our body, acidic foods form acids. They reduce the pH of fluids, including saliva, lymph, and blood, and make them more acidic. Alkaline foods increase the pH number of these fluids and make them alkaline. For general comparison, the 'standard' pH in human saliva is between 7.3 and 7.4. However, most people have less pH as they are more acidic. They are drained, burnt out, and their bodies starve for balance. Muscles are fatigued quickly under the influence of acidic foods. You are forced to slow down practically, as the body cannot produce the same results as before physically. When you consume acidic foods, free radical degradation occurs, and this induces aging. Minerals and vitamins are not readily absorbed. The digestive system is thrown off balance as pleasant bacteria die. Furthermore, the intestine's functions are impaired due to the acidity as nutrients are not absorbed so quickly. Cells become saturated with toxins that cannot be extracted. The majority of the systems in the body cannot work at maximum ability. In comparison, alkaline foods are more beneficial to well-being. Eating such foods is more beneficial. They have antioxidant effects on the body. The assimilation at cellular levels is increased, and they enable the cells to function normally. Yeast and parasitic growth are decreased due to these foods. Alkaline foods encourage more restful and deeper sleep, healthy and youthful skin, and help relieve suffering from colds, flu, and headaches. These foods also promote copious physical energy. The link to cancer is a significant distinction between acidic and alkaline foods. Safe tissues are alkaline, while cancerous tissues are acidic. When oxygen combines with an acidic fluid, it forms water due to the combination with hydrogen ions. Though oxygen helps to neutralize the acid, the acid does not allow oxygen to reach the tissues. The lone oxygen atom is open to move to another cell and extend the merits of oxygen to the other cells in the tissue. At a pH of over 7.4, cancer tissues become dormant. Studies have shown that, at pH 8.5, healthy tissues live while cancerous tissues die. There are many benefits to an alkalized diet, apart from preventing cancer. To maintain good health, balanced body chemistry must also be used - this is highly necessary for maintaining a healthy lifestyle. Too much acidic foods cause what is known as 'acidosis.' They are a fundamental explanation for some diseases and particularly in persons with arthritic and rheumatic diseases that affect their joints. You simply "burn" the food as you digest it - it becomes fuel just like a combustion engine turns gasoline into energy to propel you forward. Our fuel source is important in maintaining the balance of our health and our body, but if we have acidosis and an acidic diet, our body gets bad fuel. You wouldn't bring diesel fuel into a normal vehicle, would you? You wouldn't, of course, because your body isn't any different. We generate 'ash' as a by-product when our body burns fuel. This byproduct may have several properties. They can be harmless, acidic, or alkaline - depending on the minerals in the food. This ash happens if the blood or tissue is poor in alkaline reserves. We need to build a proportion of acid and alkaline to maintain a balance to keep our body in order. The average natural ratio is four parts of alkaline to one of acid or 80-20. While we sustain these relationships, the body has extra strong disease tolerance and improved recovery, while when the balance is out of control, the opposite is true. Disease therapies should involve high alkaline foods so that acidity compensates them for the best chance of being beaten. We have high alkaline reserves if our bodies are stable so that emergency needs can be easily met only if too much acid is swallowed. However, we will deplete these reserves, and our wellbeing can suffer significantly when the ratios start falling to three to one. We can operate normally, but only if we have enough alkaline in reserve and a correct alkaline ratio and acidic foods.

Five key alkaline foods recommended by Dr. Sebi that help our bodies maintain the correct pH balance and they are:

1. Broccoli - Broccoli is one of the vegetables that we buy, but the fantastic features that contribute to circulation and fuel usage are not always recognized.

2. Spinach – By far, one of the better options for alkaline foods with nutrients well above the average is calorie spinach.

3. Avocado - I love this fruit personally, and you know it is outstanding for reduced cholesterol and cardiovascular well-being.

4. Sprouts – Sprouts provide us with many benefits, such as lowering cholesterol and helping with heart health, but they are also rich in compounds that can affect cancer-growing cells.

5. Flaxseed Oil - This oil is rich in minerals that improve joint and bone health and, by taking a tablet a day, can reduce arthritis in the short term.

Eating plenty of alkaline foods every day will allow you to restore your body's pH balance to the best possible health.

3.9. Dr. Sebi's Alkaline Diet for Diabetics While Fasting

Regular exercises, a healthy diet, a safe physical environment, and a way of life that offers the lowest possible burden are included with this lifestyle. A healthy lifestyle allows our body to sustain at the lowest possible level the acid waste material. It suggests that the alkaline diet fits the essence of the human body best. This is mainly because it allows the body to neutralize and remove acid waste. Alkaline diets can be used by people as general human food restrictions. Individuals with unique health problems and special requirements can help adjust their preferences to the principles of alkaline diets. The miraculous alkaline diet can help improve the overall health of people with diabetes. As they do in other humans, alkaline diets help enhance body chemistry and metabolism and immune system. This diet should allow diabetics to more efficiently control their blood sugar. It can also help minimize their weight gain and cardiovascular disease risk and keep their levels of cholesterol down. Besides, the alkaline diet helps to treat diabetes well, making it possible to avoid degenerative diseases for diabetics. By following an alkaline diet, diabetics, considering their health problems, can survive longer and improve their life expectancy substantially at the same time.

3.10. Some More Alkaline Foods to consume during Dr. Sebi Fasting

Find out what to eat to better your fitness (and what to avoid)! With some exceptions, the more alkaline diets that react to sweet fruits or other unique foods are great for most, such as ulcer victims, asthma, and sugar sensitivity.

To help you boost your health, take a look at this list of alkaline and acidic foods:

Higher amounts of food are less alkaline than acidic (usually more difficult to digest).

MORE ALKALINE: Best food, even good for detoxification.

A pinch of salt in the water of lemon/calamine

- Grassy Tea
- Honey (a little)
- Apple cider vinegar
- Coconut water
- Citrus fruit juice
- Further fruit juices
- Lactobacteria eat milk-free
- Farming fruits
- Sweet fruits
- Other fruits such as super mature bananas (except starchy fruits)
- Green leafy fish and vegetables
- All other crops (except two starchy veggies in the next category and three listed at the bottom of the chart)
- Flax, hemp, cocoon, and olive oil

SEMI-ALKALINE: Perfect for healthy citizens

- Tiny quantities of lactobacteria, goat's milk yogurt is best for
- dairy alone
- Blueberry
- Hot fruit and vegetables (potato, eggplant, normal banana,
- avocado, jackfruit, breadfruit)
- Ball screw nuts (in small quantity, blended or very well-chewed, not fried)
- Raw sugar

SEMI-ACID-FORMING: suitable in small amounts

- Sweetheart Theater (which is an herb, not a grain)
- Gently sprinkled vegetables (better use coconut oil) (better use
- coconut oil)
- Millet (the most alkaline grain) (the most alkaline grain)
- Other whole grain (including 100 percent bread/rice/noodles,
- maize, oats, and garlic)
- Tofu New
- Vegetables (e.g., lentils, mung beans, soy, peanut)

ACID-FORMING:

For good people, a little is not that bad.

- Grains of refined consistency (including white rice, white bread, white noodles, veggie-meat) (including white bread, white rice, white noodles, veggie-meat)

EXTREMELY ACID-FORM: Remove or minimize

- Profound fried foods
- Fish
- Poultry
- Meat
- Eggs (hardest digestible food and bad cholesterol #1 source)

Notes:

1. Dairy goods vary from one's own – good for others, bad for others.

2. Refined sugar, tea, and coffee are not difficult to digest, but they form highly acidic and deprive the body of nutrients required to consume them in liberal terms.

3. Onion, garlic, and champagne are not difficult for absorption, but the lower drums heat up and sound rather unsettling.

Step up alkaline foods for your diet and see how your health improves!

3.11. Misconceptions about Plant-Based or Alkaline Diet

The following myths and facts help you discover some "misconceptions" of a plant-based diet or alkaline diet recommended by Dr. Sebi.

1: Fake Iron, Vegetarian and Vegan diets

2: Vegetarians are not getting a lot of protein

3: You can't adopt a vegetarian diet while you are pregnant.

4: You can't follow a vegetarian diet if you're interested in sports.

5: Kids are refusing to eat vegetarian or vegan.

6: Vegan or vegetarian foods are difficult to change.

7: Vegetarians don't like animal products.

8: Vegetarian and vegan diets should also be considered.

9: Vegetarians are not getting enough protein.

10: Vegetarians are skinny, weak, about 98 pounds.

11: Vegetarians eat potatoes.

12: Vegetarians are not getting enough calcium.

13: Vegetarians cannot eat out.

14: Vegetarians eat fish.

15: Vegetarianism is a fad of a new age.

16: Vegetarians are deluded into living forever.

3.12. Acidic Foods to Avoid

There are foods with acid reflux to avoid whether the state of hyperacidity is successfully controlled. It is necessary for the pH level to be healthy (potential hydrogen) is balanced in the body, i.e., acid and alkaline.

Since the body appears to build acid to become more acidic over time, it is important to have an alkaline diet covering various green vegetables and fruits. Broccoli, cantaloupe, almonds, apple vinegar, celery, dried dates, figs, lemon, lime, raisins, mangoes, melons, papaya, peanuts, algae, and watermelon can also be contained in alkaline items. Whilst lemon is a citrus fruit, once consumed, its properties change to high alkaline levels. Lemons are perfect for the acid crisis.

3.13. Maintain a healthy body with Dr. Sebi Fasting

Besides keeping away from food during a fasting window of the day, follow Dr. Sebi's guidelines to eat during the eating time slots. Also, stay hydrated and workout to stay fresh and mindful.

Eat more new vegetables and fruit

We know we have fruits and vegetables that are good. Some are called alkaline diets. They're not all handfuls. Even certain fruits and vegetables that are acidic are considered alkaline foods in their natural state. Among them are lemons, lime, and grapefruits. Alkaline food produces alkaline ash, which, when metabolized by the liver, neutralizes acid ash within the body. The secret to our health is a high alkaline diet. When acid removes calcium and other neutralizing nutrients, high acidity allows our bones and other joints to collapse. We should, thus, have a high intake of that form of alkaline food. We would restore our health if we did.

Physical workout

Daily exercise lets a person get healthier and works well for the mind and body. It also serves to ensure that our body has a sufficient supply of oxygen. It also helps you digest properly and promotes food habits that are good.

Drink plenty of water

It is much better when you drink alkaline water. Besides eating a high-alkaline diet, we should still consume lots of water. Yet, we need to learn that alkalizing our water is better. This we call alkaline water. Yeah, it's known for our well-being. You will accept that there is little attractiveness of a diet called alkaline. This is sometimes called an alkaline acid diet or an alkaline acid diet. It is a diet that emphasizes the eating of vegetables and fresh fruit. While it differs considerably from what other people eat, the alkaline diet is not as daunting as the label makes it appear. It relies on the consumption of a few processed airplanes or livestock. The idea is really simple. You have to eat ingredients that you know are healthy for your body, such as salads and fresh leafy vegetables, and skip products that do not contain alcohol, yeast, unhealthy grains, or sugar. You have to eat something safe for your body. An analysis is lighter than this simple breakdown, but the number of alkaline fruits, vegetables, and alkaline juices and waters that you drink needs to be optimized. This shows the alkaline food division into acidic foods by

80/20. The ratio you want is that. If it seems too complicated, don't worry, because it isn't. When properly digested, some of the foods we consume are either alkaline or acidic. Acid is present in fish, cereals, seafood, shellfish, poultry, salt, and milk, all of which are common in the Western diet. This is not necessarily valid, but you can consume more alkaline foods, such as fresh fruits and vegetables. We have very alkaline blood as a consequence, but with normal pH levels from 7.35 to 7.45. You should eat a diet that expresses the pH level of your body, and that is very alkaline, and that was for our ancestors. The predominant cause for this is that most have never known of an alkaline diet or the body's alkaline acid equilibrium. Holistic doctors and nutritionists still promote even this diet as this therapy method is deemed necessary to stay healthy and prevent diseases such as cancer.

On the other hand, most conventional doctors don't believe or support the alkaline diet. How is one meant to eat alkaline food? Some say that chronic illnesses can benefit from an alkaline diet. There are currently a few medical reports to endorse this particular diet, although most of the foods it requires you to eat are healthy foods accepted by most doctors. People who don't feel well when eating a diet low in carbohydrates or high in protein can benefit from this diet. It may also benefit people who live difficult lives and eat so many acidic items. Talking to the doctor before sticking to a diet, for instance, is also a smart practice.

Chapter 4: Dr. Sebi Recipes to Relish While Fasting

In this chapter, we will be stating few amazing recipes that can be relished during the eating time slots while following Dr. Sebi Fasting for healing, detoxification and weight-loss. These recipes are formulated using Dr. Sebi's Guidelines.

4.1. Dr. Sebi's Watermelon Refresher

Ingredients:

- Zest and juice of 1 key lime
- 2 cups soft-jelly coconut water
- 4 cups cubed watermelon
- Date sugar to taste

Directions:

1. In a blender or food processor, put the key lime juice, watermelon and zest and blend well to form a smooth mixture.

2. With the date sugar, make the mixture sweet. Remember that the taste is watered down by adding the soft-jelly coconut water,

3. Serve 1/3 coconut soft-jelly water and 2/3 watermelon combination in a big glass. Mix well and relish!

4.2. Kamut Breakfast Porridge

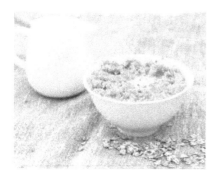

Ingredients:

- 1 cup (7 ounces) Kamut

- 3 3/4 cups homemade walnut milk or soft-jelly coconut milk

- 1/2 teaspoon sea salt

- One tablespoon coconut oil

- Four tablespoons agave syrup

Directions:

1. Blend the Kamut till you have about 1 1/4 cups of cracked Kamut on a high-speed blender or food processor.

2. Mix the crushed Kamut, walnut or coconut milk, and sea salt in a medium saucepan and whisk to mix.

3. Bring to a boil over high temperature, then reduce heat to medium-low and simmer for around 10 minutes, stirring periodically, until it thickens to your taste.

4. Stir in the coconut oil and agave syrup, then remove from the sun. If required, garnish with fresh fruit, and enjoy your Kamut porridge!

4.3. The Best Fritter Zucchini Ever

Ingredients:

- 1 Lb. of zucchini,
- 1 egg rubbed and drained
- 1 tablespoon of fresh Italian parsley
- 1/2 cup almond meal with 1/2 cup goat cheese, sea salt crumbled and black soil
- 1/2 tablespoon red pepper flakes, smashed
- Two spoonful of olive oil

Directions:

1. Blend all of the items in a blender, except for the olive oil. And place in the Refrigerator for thirty min.

2. Add the oil over a moderate flame to a non-stick frying pan; collect the heaped oil Combination of spoonsful of zucchini in hot oil.

3. Cook for 3 to 4 minutes. To suck up any extra oil, move it to a paper towel. Serve and have enjoyed!

4.4. Easy Tuna Mornay Magic

Ingredients:

- 1 chopped onion
- 2 large fresh beaten eggs, optional (this help thicken and set the casserole, but aren't necessary)
- 1 1/2 Tbsp fresh or dried parsley or chives
- 2 drained cans of tuna in olive oil or spring water
- 2 cups steamed cauliflower florets
- 1 Tbsp coconut flour, salt, and black pepper to taste

- 1/3 cup dairy-free cheese substitute, optional (1 cup of Brazil nuts and 2 cloves of garlic well blended in a food processor works a treat on the Paleo diet) raw salt and black pepper to taste.
- 1 cup coconut milk 1/2 tsp garlic flakes (optional, I only add this if not using Brazil nut and garlic topping below)

Directions:

1. Heat oven to 375F (180C). Grease with coconut or olive oil a 9-inch casserole dish

2. In a wide bowl, put all the ingredients except the cheese. Toss once mixed properly.

3. Move to a presentable casserole dish and scatter over the top with the cheese blend. Once baked, the blend will look amazing and taste delicious.

4. Bake for 35-45 minutes.

5. Sprinkle with additional parsley or herbs.

It tastes sweet, both cold and hot. Making sure it's cooled in the lunch box.

4.5. Creamy Sun-Dried Tomato Dressing

Ingredients:

- ¼ tsp Italian Seasoning

- ¼ cup Hemp Hearts*

- 2 cups Filtered Water

- 1 tbsp High-Quality Balsamic Vinegar

- ½ cup Sun-dried Tomatoes

- 1 Fresh clove Garlic

Directions:

1. Add all the ingredients to a mixer and blend them at high speed for 45-60 seconds roughly. Serve as per requirement. Place the remaining for one week at max in the Refrigerator.

Conclusion

This divisive and stringent diet focused on plants was established by the late Dr. Sebi. Proponents say that, when combined with specific dietary supplements, the risk of disease is decreased. Dr. Sebi felt nausea caused by mucus and acidity. He indicated that the intake of certain foods and the removal of others could detoxify the body, producing an alkaline atmosphere that could minimize the disease's risk and symptoms. The diet of Dr. Sebi is not officially recognized, and no scientific evidence remains that it is possible to prevent or discuss medical conditions. In certain conditions, plant-based diets can boost health, but Dr. Sebi's diet does not have enough vital nutrients to keep the body balanced. The Dr. Sebi diet requires a person to consume purely herbal food. His divisive health claims, including AIDS and leukemia, are clarified by necrology. In 1993, these and related accusations led to a complaint, which concluded with Dr. Sebi's company's order to stop issuing those claims. Dr. Sebi is confirmed to have died in 2016 while in police custody. Dr. Sebi assumed that the Western solution to sickness was inadequate. He assumed the disease was caused by acidity and mucus, such as bacteria and viruses. The fact that disease can only exist in acidic conditions is one of the main factors behind the diet. To prevent or eradicate sickness, the diet seeks to preserve an alkaline state in the body. It is also possible to adopt Dr. Sebi's diet when fasting. This book covered all of Dr. Sebi Fasting's related facets extensively.

Dr. Sebi Herbal Treatments and Cures

A brief guide to learn about herbal remedies for cure of many diseases

Introduction

Dr. Sebi is a botanist, herbalist, biochemist, and pathologist. He has explored herbs and has directly encountered them in Central America, South and North America, the Caribbean, and Africa. Using an alkaline diet and herbs that are thoroughly rooted through over 30 years of study and practice, he has established a process and system for the treatment of the human body.

Alfredo Bowman, also known as Dr. Sebi, was born on November 26, 1933, in Ilanga, Honduras, Spain. Dr. Sebi is a guy who is self-teaching. Together with the help of his grandmother, his early days of finding and trailing along the river and in the forest provided Sebi with the basis for his later life to stay true to the facts.

Sebi arrived in the United States as a self-educated guy suffering with diabetes, hypertension, impotence, and obesity. After failed experiments with Western doctors and new medications, Sebi was conveyed to an herbalist in Mexico. He started to produce natural plant cell food compounds appropriate for intercellular replication and the redevelopment of the cells that make up the human body, generating important healing effects from all his illnesses. Dr. Sebi has invested more than 30 years of his life creating a modern approach that can only be accomplished by years of clinical experience.

Motivated by personal knowledge and his own healing experience, he started to articulate his own positive clinical experience that gave rise to Dr. Sebi's Cell Food.

Majority of modern diseases and their causes

Before we jump through the significances, let us reflect what an illness is. In the operation & growth of a human person, animals, or plants, sickness is an abnormality or ailment that is not linked to an external or physical disability. Specific signs and indications also affect them, like a specific region of the body.

When people hear of the world's worse illnesses, their minds are capable of jumping to fast-acting and irrepressible ones that also draw notice. In fact, however, many of these types of illnesses are not acknowledged among the prevalent causes of death in the world.

Even more astonishingly, all of the world's worse ailments are, perhaps, inevitable. The non-preventable factors include where a person lives, the quality of clinical insurance, and precautionary health services. But still, there are steps everyone can take in order to reduce their jeopardy.

Chapter 1-Natural Components and Remedies Care

1.1 Treatment for medicinal aging

Life expectancy has risen from about 41 years in several developing countries to about 80. In the early 1950s. The percentage of older citizens (sixty-five years & over) in our societies is also growing. The greying of our culture carries a growing burden of illness & irreversible aging-related dependence. Aging is linked with a gradual reduction in neurological activity and an enhanced risk of death, coronary failure, elevated blood pressure, diabetes mellitus, hypertension, osteoporosis, etc. In assessing the length and quality of a healthy existence and even in combating infectious disorders, behavioral variables such as exercise or diet play a crucial role. While several aging hypotheses have been proposed over the years, there is no straightforward reason for aging. Genetic factors are undeniably significant, yet of all the biochemical causes for aging, the oxidative stress hypothesis remains the most widely supported concept (Beckman and Ames 1998; Harman 1992). This hypothesis postulates that aging is induced by the accumulation of irreversible damage, i.e. oxidative stress produced by oxidation arising from the association between reactive oxygen species and cell DNA, protein and lipid components. Although it is claimed that the aging phase itself is not attributable to oxidative stress, common chronic age-related disorders have also exacerbated oxidative stress. In plants, antioxidants can contribute to at least some of their reputed medicinal outcomes.

1.2 Care based on herbals

Herbal medicine is "the knowledge, theories, and approaches based on indigenous philosophies, concepts, and connections to multiple ethnicities, used for the treatment, assessment, improvement or cure of mental & physical disease for health protection and prevention." Herbal medicine has several distinct mechanisms, and the theory is regulated by the climate of each case, usually, irrespective of the actual sickness or ailment that the patient welfares from, the attention remains on the individual's physical wellbeing, and the utilization of herbs is a decisive feature of many traditional medication systems.

In a systematic approach to contemporary medical treatment (TCM), traditional Chinese medicine has been a noteworthy illustration of how classical & contemporary expertise is implemented. TCM has a past of over 3000 years. The book "The Devine Farmer's Classic of Herbalism" was written in China over 2000 years ago, and it is the world's oldest recorded herbal text. The documented and methodically collected herbal statistics, however, have grown into numerous herbal pharmacopeias, and there are many specific herbal monographs.

Treatment and care, viewed in the sense of the Yin-yang combination, are focused on a positive perception of the illness and the effects of the disorder. Yin portrays femininity, soil, and ice, whereas yang describes the sky, masculinity, and heat. Yin and Yang's behaviors affect the relationships of the world's five elements: wood, water, metal, earth, and fire. TCM practice intention is to control the degrees of Yang & Yin across 12 apogees that bring energy (Qi) through a body and direct it. TCM is a mounting method internationally, and it is used both to boost well-being and to reduce and prevent illnesses. TCM involves many practices, but the main aspect is conventional treatments and natural elements.

Clinical medicine has been transformed in many areas of the world during the last 100 years with the invention & widespread production of chemically generated medicines. Large portions of the populace in developed nations, though, also depend on conventional practitioners and natural primary care therapies. Up to 90 percent of people in Africa and 70% in India rest on natural therapies to meet their medical requirements. In China, conventional medicine refers to around 40 percent of all health care given, and more than ninety percent of public hospitals have traditional medicine units. However, the usage of herbal medications is not exclusive to developing nations, and over the past two decades, with the growing use of ethnobotanicals, the general interest of herbal remedies has greatly increased in industrialized countries.

The most common explanations for the usage of natural drugs are because they are more effective, resonate more generally with the consumer's lifestyle, alleviate worries regarding the harmful effects of chemical (synthetic) medicines, meet the need for more customized health treatment, and support a more systematic tactic by the public to health records. Encouraging human well-being and curing viral ailments and avoiding life-threatening conditions is the principal application of herbal medicines. The usage of natural treatments, however, is growing as current treatment is inadequate in the clinical treatment of advanced tumors and new infectious diseases, for example. Natural drugs, in contrast, are widely incorporated, not hazardous, and are healthy & safe.

The herbal treatment delivers an essential health care option, whether people are financially or medically susceptible to allopathic drugs, which are a growing global market, regardless of whether a person needs it.

Plants are currently used to treat common and crippling diseases and numerous illnesses and complications, such as heart dysfunction, prostate disorders, obesity, asthma, anxiety, and immune enhancement. Traditional natural therapies played a crucial role in China's SARS (Serious Acute Respiratory Syndrome) management and care plan in 2003. A common herbal remedy, the vine of Africans has been used to cure HIV-related indications in Africa for years. In Europe, herbal medical things are also trendy. France & Germany, the leading European countries in total trades of medicinal extracts or teas and essential oils, can be sold in pharmacies in most industrialized countries offering generic medicines.

It is necessary to grow plants and seeds and may be used in different ways and varieties, including entire herbs, teas, syrups, lavender oil, ointments, salves, rubbers, pills, and capsules containing a raw herb type powdered dried extract. Vinegar (extracts of acetic acid), alcoholic extracts, extracts of hot water (tisanes), long boiling extracts, typically bark, and roots (decoctions), and cold herbal extracts. There is a limited standard and the ingredients in an herbal invention often vary greatly across batches & suppliers.

Plant species are rich in a range of chemicals. Most are secondary metabolites of plants that contain aromatic compounds that are mostly phenols or variants of phenols combined with oxygen, such as tannins. Both of these compounds are antioxidants.

1.3 Nature-extracted analgesic agents (natural products)

Various types of natural products have been used to relieve pain conditions since the earliest recorded accounts, around 7000 years ago. These authentic items are representations of the opium poppy (Papaver soniferum) and willow tree bark (Salix spp.). It was not until the nineteenth century that these chemicals were extracted from complex compounds and were thought to produce the results necessary. The known origins of such compounds have been studied in detail. Additional analgesic compounds have been derived from natural resources during the last several decades, resulting in various molecular groups and modes of action. The more modern focus in opioid research activities has been in plants or other natural remedies related to in ancient ethnopharmacological and ethnobotanical literature. These studies and documents identify better pharmaceutical ingredients than have been used widely in pain treatment. The underlying knowledge of the diverse pain signaling mechanisms in the nervous system has been a significant factor that has demonstrated the importance of finding new compounds to relieve pain. Nociceptive development includes various types of receptors, enzymes, and signaling pathways. The identification of novel groups of compounds through natural sources will contribute to a better understanding of these pharmacological pathways. With the potential to identify new medicines with favorable pharmacological attributes (i.e. no risks to wellbeing, no opportunity to become addicted), natural products are therefore highly promising for the future of drug development, especially in the treatment of pain and possibly opioid addictions.

1.4 Anti-inflammatory activity in natural products

Multiple inflammatory diseases are widespread in the world's aging population. The downside to adverse responses and prescribing rates are the clinically administered anti-inflammatory medications (in biologic drugs). Alternatively, these therapies are medicinal remedies and natural resources that show great potential for the production and manufacture of biologically active lead compounds for the treatment of inflammatory diseases. Since ancient times, natural remedies and leading pharmaceuticals have been used to cure inflammation and other diseases. The metabolites listed belong to different chemicals such as steroids, alkaloids, polyphenolics, and terpenoids that play a vital role in anti-inflammatory properties. Research into natural goods and substances obtained from environmental assets has also grown in recent years owing to their connotation in the discovery of medicines. In plants that are of immense value to humans, numerous compounds with antifungal action against various strains of fungi have been identified. Those molecules can be used as a guide to making better molecules.

1.5 Mediated plant antifungal agents

A modern continuum of human fungal infections is growing as a result of increased cancer, AIDS, and patients with a weakened immune system. The increased application of antifungal agents has also resulted in the creation of modern drug tolerance. New types of antifungal agents to treat fungal infections appear to be classified.

1.6 Heart attack by ischemia or by the cardiac malfunction

Ischemic heart disease is a chronic lung pain or depression condition where insufficient oxygen in the heart is present. This disorder most frequently occurs from exertion or distress as the heart needs a larger supply of blood. Ischemic cardiac disease is expected in the United States and is a major cause of death internationally, also recognized as a coronary heart attack.

As particles of blood cholesterol appear to pile up on the walls of the arteries to supply blood to the heart, ischemic heart attack happens. Deposits, which are called plaques, may gradually form. These deposits, which end up restricting the supply of blood, shorten the lungs. This reduction in blood flow reduces the amount of oxygen supplied to the heart muscle.

Symptoms and symptoms of ischemic heart disease can slowly develop as the arteries become mildly blocked, or if the artery is spontaneously blocked, they may occur quickly. In certain individuals with cardiovascular disorder, there are also no signs, but some may feel shortness of breath and extreme chest pain (angina) that may lead to the risk of a heart attack.

Fortunately, ischemic heart disease may be effectively treated through dietary enhancements. And further, by adopting heart-healthy habits, such as cooking, low-sodium eating, a low-fat diet, getting more active, not smoking, and sustaining a healthy diet, you will decrease the chances of ischemic heart failure.

Severe coronary injury can be incurred by ischemic heart failure if left unchecked. Cardiac injury may cause heart loss and pain, as well as life-threatening harm.

Causes

Induced by inadequate blood flow to one of the oxygen-pumping blood vessels, ischemic heart failure (coronary arteries). While blood pressure is lowered, the muscle of the heart does not get the amount of oxygen it needs to function properly.

Cardiac ischemia may develop slowly; as plaque builds up over time, or when an artery is totally blocked, it may occur quickly. For this reason, ischemic heart failure more often arises in people of atherosclerosis (plaque build-up on the coronary artery walls), coronary artery spasm, blood clots, or severe diseases that intensify the central need for oxygen.

What risk aspects have heart ischemia implications?

The risk of developing ischemic heart failure is increased by multiple factors. Not all with risk factors receive ischemic heart failure. Risk indicators for cardiac ischemia include:

- High cholesterol level in the blood
- History of familial cardiac problems
- High level of Triglycerides in blood
- Hypertension
- The body high in fats
- Diabetes Mellitus
- Tobacco and many other applications
- No exercise or physical movement

1.7 STDs

Sexually transmitted diseases (STDs) are viruses that, by sexual contact, flow from one person to another. Parasites, bacteria, and viruses are the sources of STDs. Over 20 kinds of STDs are available, including

- The Occurrence of Chlamydia
- Genital herpes
- Gonorrhea
- AIDS/HIV
- Trichomoniasis
- Syphilis
- HPV

In certain cases, STDs also impact both men and women, though women may be more concerned with health problems. The child may have severe health problems while the mother is pregnant with an STD.

STDs caused by bacteria or by parasites may be treated with antibiotics. STDs triggered by an illness are not treated, but medications may still aid with the symptoms of maintaining the disease under control.

The Occurrence of Chlamydia

Chlamydia trachomatis, a bacterium, also triggers unchecked genital, oral, or vaginal sex to produce chlamydia. An individual may get it from the vaginal fluid or sperm of an infected person. It may also be spread by genital interaction from an affected human to another, even if there is no sexual interaction.

Genitals Herpes

Genital herpes is a common sexually transmitted disease or infection induced by HSV (herpes simplex virus). The key source of the disorder is sexual intimacy.

Gonorrhea

The leading cause of Gonorrhea is the sexually transmitted bacterium that contaminates both men and women. It usually affects the rectum, throat, or urethra. In women, it can also influence the cervix. The extent of the infection is through genital, vaginal, or anal intercourse.

Aids

Acquired immunodeficiency syndrome is a life-threatening and chronic HIV mediated illness. In order to fight disease and cancer, it damages the immune system by interfering with the body's potential.

Trichomoniasis

A protozoan parasite called Trichomonas vaginalis is the cause of this common, sexually transmitted illness.

Syphilis

Treponema Pallidum induces syphilis. There is an illness that is viral. The leading cause of infection is sexual intercourse, mucous membranes, or abrasions, or superficial skin wounds.

HPV

The human papillomavirus enters the human body through a small tear or a cut in the tissue. It is communicated mainly by skin-to-skin contact. About 100 HPV types are involved, influencing many areas of the body. Genital HPV is spread via anal sex, physical intercourse, or other skin-to-skin touches inside the genital region.

1.8 Cancer or Tumor

Cancer may begin anywhere inside the body. It starts as cells quickly replicate and fill the amount of normal cells. That makes it hard for the body to work the way it should.

Any people may be willing to handle cancer well. Because of cancer therapy, more individuals have longer lives than ever before.

We'll chat here about what the causes of cancer are. Not only is cancer a single ailment.

There are many tumors present. This isn't about any single illness. Cancer can begin in the breast, in the lungs, the colon, or in the blood. In basic ways, cancers are similar but vary in the way they develop and propagate.

Why does cancer appear the same?

Our cells do have some tasks to do in our bodies. Standard cells differentiate in an orderly manner. They die and fresh cells grow as they are stretched out or injured. As the cells start spreading out of balance, cancer arises. New cells are continuing to grow and become cancer cells. They clutch off normal cells. Which produces problems in the region of the body where cancer starts.

Sometimes, cancer cells are spread to other areas of the body. For example, lung cancer cells may move to the bones and spread. As cancer cells spread, metastasis is named (meh-TAS-uh-sis). Therefore, once lung disease extends to the bones, it is considered a tumor of the lungs. Cancer cells tend to be like doctors, mostly in the bones, just like the lungs. If it originates from the bones, it is referred to as bone cancer.

What are certain cancers?

The development and distribution of such tumors are fast. The other will inevitably arise. They respond to counseling in many ways often. Some cancer forms are best treated by surgery; others react favorably to chemotherapy. Usually, 2 or 3 techniques are used to yield maximum performance.

Maybe the specialist would prefer to figure out what type of cancer it is. People struggling with cancer need care that fits their kind of cancer.

What are these sorts of tumors?

Multiple tumors are formed by a lump called a growing tumor. Lumps, though, are not inherently a disorder. Health care staff pull out a section of the swelling to search to see if there is cancer. The word assigned to non-cancer bumps or lumps is Benign. Cancer-causing lumps are called malignant.

Tumors such as leukemia (blood cancer) do not build tumors. They expand in the body's blood cells or in other cells.

There is anxiety raging inside you as you are notified you have cancer. It's so difficult to think about something other than sickness at the onset. This is the first thing you do every morning to consider or chat about. I want patients with cancer to realize that they're feeling stronger. Worrying over cancer encourages you to cope with all the many thoughts that you have. Note, it is common to get irritated.

What is caused by cancer?

By sustained gene destruction, cancer may be caused. The risk or response to the cancer-causing agent can be due to these variations.

The cancer-causing compounds are known as carcinogens. The chemical portion may be carcinogens, such as those chemicals that burn cigarettes. Cancer may also be caused by viral, biological, or genetic causes.

We should keep in mind, however, that we do not assign the illness to a source in most cancer situations.

We can categorize risk factors for cancer into approximately the following groups:

- Environmental sensitivity to U.V. radiation & radon, & small particulates

- Internal or biological features, counting gender, age, defects that are genetically inherited, and skin type.

- Features linked to lifestyle.

- Occupational features include carcinogens such as certain pesticides, asbestos, and unclean materials

Factors linked to lifestyle which source cancer comprise:

- Alcohol

- U.V. radiations

- Tobacco

- Several factors are connected to food, such as barbecue-generated polyaromatic hydrocarbons & nitrites.

Some cancer-causing aspects linked to the living atmosphere and work comprise:

- Hydrocarbons that are polynuclear (e.g., benzopyrene), and asbestos fibers

- Pitch & tar

- Certain toxic plastic chemicals (e.g., vinyl chloride)

- Certain compounds made of metal

Bacteria & viruses can encourage cancer:

- HCV, HBV (hepatitis virus causing hepatitis)

- Helicobacter pylori (blamed for gastritis)

- Epstein-Barr virus (herpes virus triggering lymphoid gland inflammation).

- HPV (human papillomavirus, papillomavirus inducing modifications, for example, in the cervical cells)

Cancer through radiation:

- Non-ionized radiation (U.V. radiation from the sun)

- Radiation ionizing (e.g., surface radon, X-rays)

Some medicines may elevate cancer jeopardy:

- Some hormones

- Some lump antineoplastic agents

- Medicinal products which trigger an immune shortage

Genetic predisposition plays a significant part in developing the condition in 5 – 10 percent of breast cancer.

1.9 Diabetes Mellitus

Diabetes mellitus, commonly referred to as diabetes, is a metabolic disorder which causes high levels of blood sugar. The hormone insulin transfers glucose from the blood into cells for energy intake or application. Diabetes suggests that the body either does not have adequate insulin or does not consume the insulin it produces properly.

Owing to untreated high blood sugar diabetes, the muscles, nerves, liver, and other organs would be damaged.

There are numerous types of diabetes:

- Type 1 diabetes occurs as the body becomes insulin resistant, and blood sugar builds up.
- Type 2 diabetes, which is an infectious state. The body's immune system destroys the pancreatic cells, where insulin is produced. What triggers an attack is not evident. Around 10 percent of persons living with diabetes have this form of the condition.
- Prediabetes usually develops when the amount of blood sugar in the bloodstream is elevated than average, but not severe enough for type 2 diabetes to be detected.
- Blood sugar in gestational diabetes is elevated during birth. This kind of diabetes is induced by insulin-suppressing hormones released by the placenta.

Diabetes mellitus is not synonymous with a rare condition named diabetes insipidus, although it has a similar name. This is natural, for the kidneys drain a great deal of body moisture.

There are signs, causes, and medications for each diabetes condition.

Prompts of Diabetes

There are distinct factors of some form of diabetes.

- Type 1 diabetes

A variety of biochemical and lifestyle-related causes contribute to type 2 diabetes. Being overweight or obese often enhances the risk. Carrying additional fats, especially in the abdomen, makes it possible for the cells to be extremely immune to the blood glucose impact of insulin.

The disease is spreading throughout nations. Chromosomes that boost their risk of having type 2 diabetes and becoming overweight are expressed by family members.

- Type 2 diabetes

Healthcare experts are confused regarding what is responsible for type 1 diabetes. The immune system unintentionally targets and eliminates the insulin-producing beta-cells in the pancreas for no purpose.

In certain people, genes may play a part. Even a virus will set off a strain on the immune system.

- Gestational Diabetes

Gestational diabetes is the result of increases in hormone levels when breastfeeding. The placenta produces hormones that make the cells of a pregnant woman less vulnerable to the effects of insulin. This may induce elevated amounts of blood sugar during conception.

Women who are overweight before birth or who have extra weight after pregnancy are more prone to develop gestational diabetes.

1.10 The Bottom Line

From the early days of civilization, herbs, fruits, plants, and ethnobotanicals have been used and are now used worldwide for health elevation and disease deterrence. The foundation is created by plants and natural springs in modern medicine today and applies principally to the industrial drug formulations produced today. About 25 percent of the world's prescription drugs are manufactured from plants. Considering that plants are sometimes exploited in health treatment, rather than medicines. For certain individuals, their desired method of care is herbal therapy. Herbs are used as an adjunct drug to regular pharmaceuticals and others. In several developed countries, however, conventional medicine, a central component of which is herbal medicine, is the only type of healthcare accessible or efficient.

Chapter 2: Uses of Different Herbs by Dr. Sebi to Cure Harpies, Diabetes and Other Diseases

2.1 Diabetes

This recommends that the blood sugar level often mentioned to as blood glucose, will be too high if you have diabetes. A hormone called insulin is usually used to help renovate food into energy. When a person has diabetes, his or her body either does not have insulin or cannot tolerate use insulin. It may cause major health difficulties, renal failure, heart disorder, and blindness if diabetes is not managed. By maintaining blood sugar under a safe amount, living healthily, and becoming actively active, diabetes may be controlled. You have to change your way of dining. Type 2 diabetes is mainly something of a dietary disorder since it is widely known and can be regulated through dietary change. It's safer to consume a plant-based alkaline diet. According to Dr. Sebi, the body is most likely to be in an acidic condition and the source of all diseases is mucus. Where the disease is involved, there would be excessive mucus. In his method, Dr. Sebi helped millions of people with diabetes, and his death did nothing to improve this; he left behind medical curing strategies for diabetes. You will learn from his hypothesis about what he really believes about this lethal illness in order to eliminate diabetes from the earth's land; here is the entire description of Dr. Sebi's diabetes solution.

2.2 Normal rehabilitations for Type 2 diabetes

Type 2 diabetes (also known as diabetes mellitus) results from the domino effect of poor activity, too many incorrect foods, insomnia, mental tiredness, insomnia, biology, and contaminants. In addition to their traditional treatments, individuals with type 2 diabetes more commonly turn to herbal therapy to control their condition. A great approach to supplement diabetes care is through alternative treatments by the usage of herbal medicines. However, combining plants, supplements, and medications will lead to a decrease in blood sugar levels termed hypoglycemia if applied without the appropriate instructions or directions.

The list of natural treatments for type 2 diabetes can be found below.

Barley and Fabric

Consuming fiber lowers amounts of blood sugar and insulin. The prescribed fiber consists of around 30 grams a day. Many Americans, which is not acceptable, get about 6-8 grams. Although you might prescribe fiber supplements like Metamucil, eating your vegetables is the perfect way to accomplish your target! Barley is a high-protein, high-fiber grain with ample of data to support its involvement in raising levels of blood sugar, cholesterol, insulin, and general inflammation. Barley does not need to be washed and can typically cook with only a little water and salt on the top of the burner in much less than fifteen minutes.

Apple's cider vinegar

Acetic acid is the main compound in ACV and is considered liable for all of its beneficial effects. There are many approaches in using ACV that is evidence-based. By consuming two teaspoons until bedtime, you'll lower your blood sugar. Best still, 1-2 tbsp. of ACV used for cooking will reduce the glycemic burden of a meal rich in carbohydrates. It is advised for patients to either take ACV alone before a meal or combine it into salad dressings and teas.

Zing

Besides, people living with diabetes are found to suppress zinc. Zinc supplementation tests have shown that it can reduce A1C and blood sugar levels, have antioxidant activity, lower blood sugar, and even have improved diabetes-related management risks. Solid zinc doses will avoid the ingestion of additional minerals such as copper, so make sure to ask for the necessary dosing instructions.

Chromium

Chromium is primarily found in the brewer's yeast; glucose tolerance is affected by chromium deficiency. The evidence confirms chromium for lower blood sugar and A1C levels. But be vigilant if this supplement makes you suffer from kidney disease.

Aloe Vera

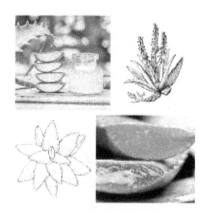

Due to its laxative influence, Aloe vera sap is known. Therefore, make sure to get the gel juice! There is growing evidence that gel, which is also the mucilaginous substance within the leaves, is being used. Make sure any drug you buy is aloin-free or anthraquinone-free to save yourself in the wash.

Cinnamon

A medically beneficial indulgence that helps to reduce cholesterol and blood sugar levels.

Berberine

New research reinforces that smaller levels of hba1c and blood sugar are used. Be mindful of how this herb can conflict with conventional medical metabolism and must never be taken while breastfeeding.

Fenugreek

Fenugreek reduces levels of cholesterol and hba1c. With this herb, one's urine can always smell like maple syrup, but this is not harmful.

Nopal

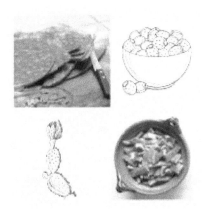

Help for reducing the amount of blood sugar.

Gymnema

The analysis is starting to catch up with its therapeutic use, indicating advantages as an alternative to the production of conventional glucose metabolism pharmaceuticals and insulin levels.

2.3 Natural and Herbal treatments

It is stated that many common spices and herbs have decreased blood sugar properties, making them suitable for people with or at high risk of type 2 diabetes.

In recent years, many medical studies have been performed that indicate possible correlations between herbal therapies and enhanced control of blood glucose, leading to expanded use of these more 'natural' drugs in people suffering from diabetes to help cure their disease.

What are natural remedies available?

Of some animals, anti-diabetic properties occur. Any of such plants are here:

- Cinnamon
- Bitter melon
- Aloe vera
- Ginger
- Fenugreek
- Okra
- Bilberry extract

Additional therapies of plants

Plants and herb derivatives mentioned below have historically been used by indigenous people in the treatment of diabetes in the places where they develop.

Coccinia, Indica

In the Indian subcontinent, Coccinia indica is often recognized and widely cultivated as the 'ivy gourd'. Insulin-mimetic properties have been shown to be widely used in ayurvedic therapies (i.e., it imitates the insulin function).

Allium Sativum

Micro-circulatory effects and antioxidant properties are known to give Allium sativum, more commonly referred to as garlic. The results have been promising, but few studies have directly linked allium to insulin and blood glucose levels. Allium can cause increased secretion, reduced blood glucose levels, and slow insulin degradation.

Ginseng

For several different plant forms, Ginseng is a common term. A drop in fasting blood glucose has been reported in some studies using American ginseng. Among the varieties are ginseng from Korea, ginseng from Siberia, ginseng from America, and ginseng from Japan. The herb, particularly the Panax species, is celebrated as 'healing-all' in certain countries. Further long-term studies are needed to confirm the efficacy of ginseng, as is the case for many of the herbs used worldwide in the treatment of diabetics.

Ficus Carica

Fig-leaf or Ficus Carican is well-known as a diabetic cure in Spain and South-West

Europe, but the active ingredient is uncertain. Any animal research indicates that glucose absorption is facilitated by the fig-leaf.

Momordica Charantia

It is ancestral to many countries in Africa, South America, and Asia. This, marketed as charantia, is also known as bitter melon or karolla, or karela. The herb can be treated in several forms and can assist in the production of insulin, glucose oxidation, and other processes for people with diabetes. They have an instant influence on blood sugar levels as well.

Gymnema Sylvestre

Gymnema Sylvestre is also used in Ayurvedic herbal medicine. The plant grows in Southern and Central India's tropical forests and has been related to a significant reduction in blood glucose. Some animal studies have also recorded an improvement in beta-cell function and islet cell regeneration.

Opuntia Streptacantha

In the arid regions where it breeds, it is generally known as the prickly-pear cactus.

Mexican desert inhabitants have traditionally employed the plant to control glucose. Some of the properties of the plant can influence intestinal glucose uptake, and significant decreases in HbA1c and postprandial glucose and HbA1c have been reported in animal studies.

Ocimum sanctum

It is a herb used in common medicine that is generally referred to as holy basil. A driven clinical trial showed a positive influence on fasting and postprandial glucose, and experts expect that the herb will increase beta-cell functionality and facilitate the mechanism of insulin secretion.

Again, to verify that the prickly pear cactus is a good alternative for the care of diabetes patients, long-term clinical studies are required.

Silybum Marianum

It is sometimes referred to as milk thistle, a family member of asters. Silymarin includes significant concentrations of flavonoids and antioxidants, both of which may have a beneficial effect on insulin resistance. There is little knowledge of the importance of Silybum marianum in glycemic control.

Some plants are also being investigated and may have positive effects for diabetes patients. Several of them are listed below:

- Cinnamomym Tamala
- Curry
- Pterocarpus marsupium
- Berberine
- Eugenia jambolana
- Vinca rosea

- Gingko
- Solanum torvum
- Phyllanthus amarus

2.4 Herpes

People also want to hear what Dr. Sebi says regarding the prevention of herpes, what his herpes cure is, and whether the usage of Dr. Sebi's herpes care drugs is possible.

Dr. Sebi talked briefly regarding his thoughts on diseases and what he believes is necessary to reverse such pathogens. With regards to recovery, he embraced a medicinal and cellular approach, and herpes was no different. Dr. Sebi talked about treating herpes in many lectures and seminars. We'll discuss this in the later section.

2.5 The Herpes Treatment of Dr. Sebi

Why does Dr. Sebi have the ability for herpes to be cured? Most simply, by the cleaning, nourishing, and detoxifying of the body. Here are the treatments focused on Dr. Sebi's soothing method.

- Prevent the position of acidic foods in the body.
- Alkaline plants prefer to be used to wash out pollutants and acids from the body (which often raises oxygen to cells).
- Feeding the body's nutrients to restore, reconstruct, and develop on a cellular scale.

Detoxification has been at the root of herpes virus destruction of the body-no another route can have the optimal effects.

2.6 Dr. Sebi's herpes medications

One might begin with a little kit for herpes cleaning. It is made up of Bio-Ferro, Chelation 2, and Viento.

- Chelation 2: extracts contaminants, mucus, fats, and cleanses the intestine. It's a chelator, like.
- Viento: This is for purifying, rejuvenating, and revitalizing cells. The central nervous, lymphatic, renal, and respiratory systems are triggered by it.
- Iron Plus and Bio Ferro: nourishing and cleaning the blood by supplying the bone with iron.

2.7 The Herpes Healing Approaches

Fasting and Herbs

During this time, you can do it quickly and you can opt to take herbs to sanitize the body and raise the consumption of iron. Dr. Sebi has confirmed on several occasions the importance of iron in healing. You may eat spices, drink green juices and water during this time.

Herbs and Diet of Alkaline

For herpes recovery, an alkaline diet is needed. Dr. Sebi emphasized the importance of this and how important it is to remove 'blood and starch,' in reference to animal flesh, including both animal species, seafood, and starchy foods, as he describes it. However, it is important to go past this when it comes to herpes recovery when even some of the things on Dr. Sebi's food list or dietary guide can be avoided. Oh, and why? Only that some of the goods are better for calming than others. Dr. Sebi said the 'least dangerous' products are in his collection, so you want something as alkaline and refreshing as possible. Fasting was also thought to be such an essential element in Dr. Sebi's recovery-it enabled the body to break from the consumption of mucus-producing foods and acids; washing would continue and the amount of oxygen to the cells will improve.

At this moment, consume alkaline plants, not just to aid with detox, but also to rejuvenate and recharge the body and improve immunity.

What are you going to do precisely?

1. Avoid utilizing foods that are fried.

2. Delete from the diet all acid-forming items.

3. For fasting, just take the water and herbs (if you can't incorporate green juices).

4. Instantly, after a period of quick eating, only vegetables, and fruits from the nutritional guide, which also features new green juices. In your leafy plants, green fluids are predominantly present. The less nutritious the diet is, during washing and detox, the easier and more successful the regeneration process is.

5. Even then, start consuming just stuff from the dietary guide until you have removed herpes from the body.

How long is the herpes treatment going to take?

When questioned, Dr. Sebi answered quite correctly that it depends on the degree of toxicity of the body, fluid, weight, and state of health. Everyone requires a particular stage of the exercise, and so the recovery duration varies so that the healing time changes between people.

How devoted are you?

Herpes can be detoxified from the body, but the results rely on how dedicated you are to the procedure. Herpes is not the best virus to clear since it retains residence in the central nervous system spinal cord and thus sits inactive there for a considerable period. Your body needs to basically 'wake it up' and usher it out. It is vital that the herpes virus is not accessible to the body. Indeed, an alkaline body is needed to keep the body alkaline by washing and treating the body with alkaline plants and alkaline food and fasting to get rid of herpes. Dr. Sebi's is this strategy.

Ruits, grains, and seeds ought to be removed while recovering from herpes. It is proposed to involve mangos, citrus fruits, leafy greens, and berries

Chapter 3: Dr. Sebi Diet Fundamental's and Importance of alkaline body

An alkaline diet is free of acid-containing ingredients, often referred to as electric fuel, which helps the body to cure itself. In nature, they are usually contained. They support the rise of copper, various essential vitamins and minerals, and iron, allowing a healthy and competent immune system.

An alkaline diet depends on the premise that it can promote your health by substituting acid-forming meals with alkaline ingredients. Supporters of this diet often say that dangerous ailments such as cancer will be best avoided. The concept behind an alkaline diet refers to this chapter. The alkaline diet is a.k.a the alkaline ash diet or acid-alkaline diet. Their idea is that the body's pH benefit is impaired by the meal, deciding alkalinity or acidity. Metabolism is often related to combustion and is the preparation of food for energy conversion. Both include the chemical process of breaking down a mass of solids. However, in a gradual and regulated way, the body's chemical reactions occur. An ash layer is left after artifacts are shot. Similarly, a "rock" residue called metabolic waste is left from the stuff you consume. The metabolic waste is likely to be alkaline, acidic, or neutral. This diet supporter believes metabolic waste may have a significant influence on the acidity of the body. In other terms, it makes the blood even more acidic if you ingest something that leaves acidic ash. It makes the blood even more alkaline as you consume something that leaves alkaline ash. It is believed that acidic ash renders you susceptible to bacteria and illness, according to the acid-ash hypothesis, whereas alkaline ash is considered defensive. You will 'alkalize' the body, and enhance the well-being, by choosing more alkaline foods. Beef, phosphorus, and Sulphur contain food components which leave acidic ash, while calcium, potassium, and magnesium are alkaline components. Neutral, acidic, or alkaline is what every form of food is called:

Neutral: starch, sugar, and fat of natural origin.

Alkaline: herbs, legumes, almonds, and fruit

Acids: meat, livestock, dairy products, vegetables, animal goods, grains, alcohol

The metabolic waste, or debris, left from the burning of foods will directly influence the acidity/alkalinity of the body, according to proponents of the diet policy.

The Alkaline Diet refers to a balanced diet that promotes whole-body and bone well-being by ensuring, within the body, an optimal pH equilibrium. The alkalizing forerunners it contains to enable the bones to conduct their functions of metabolic without being exhausted. The Alkaline Diet is the same nutritional pattern that allows cardiac attack, high blood pressure, stroke, diabetes, and chronic diseases to be avoided. It is a diet that is high in alkalizing minerals & plant compounds that encourage well-being.

Fed Alkaline for the Life is based on consuming the following food types, along with sufficient protein and vital fats. The diet focuses on:

- Veggies.
- Seeds & Nuts
- Fruits
- Pulses and spices (turmeric, mustard seed, ginger, cloves, etc.)
Both meals should be alkaline food for survival.

No matter what kind of food you choose, by merely balancing the consumption of alkaline and food that are acid-forming as a way of alkalizing the composition of the body, the diet will become an alkaline diet. If you follow a Keto, Mediterranean, elevated carb, vegan, vegetarian, or weight reduction lifestyle, what you need to do is use any of the fruits, nuts, veggies, and seeds that are alkaline-forming and approved in your eating plan. The practice of alkalizing mineral items to create an Alkaline Diet for life for every diet may also be beneficial.

Nearly none is more critical when it comes to increasing bone content than improving the acid-alkaline balance through an alkaline diet routine. Even if you turn and control pollutants, you would also get excessive bone damage in the long run if the acid-alkaline level is off-kilter. The main aspect of natural bone protection is an alkaline diet.

3.1 Acid-forming diets and acidity

A chronic bone condition marked by a decline in the mineral content of the tissue is osteoporosis. It's wildly normal in postmenopausal women & may significantly raise the chance of fractures. Many supporters of alkaline diets think that the body receipts alkaline minerals like calcium from the bones to balance the enzymes from the materials (acid-forming) you eat to maintain a steady blood pH.

Acid-forming diets, like the traditional Western diet, can, according to this hypothesis, trigger a decrease in bone mineral solidity. The following theory is called the 'acid-ash hypothesis'. In this hypothesis, the work of your kidneys is lacking, and this is important for acid removal and body pH control. The kidneys create bicarbonate ions that nullify the blood acids, enabling your body to regulate the pH in your blood closely. The pH of the blood is also managed by the respiratory system. When the kidney attaches bicarbonate ions to acids in the blood, the CO_2 they breathe out and the urine they piss out is produced.

The acid-ash theory is often overlooked by one of the key drivers of osteoporosis, diminishing bone protein collagen. Ironically, this collagen deficiency is closely correlated with inadequate amounts of two acids in the diet, orthosilicic acid & ascorbic acid and vitamin C. Bear in mind the mixed scientific evidence that relates dietary acid to the solidity of bone or danger of fracture. Although no connection was established in some qualitative studies, some observed a stable relationship. Scientific studies, which aim to be more specific, also found that diets that are acid-forming have no influence on the levels of calcium in the body.

These diets promote bone defense by gaining from synaptic regeneration and stimulating the hormone IGF-1, which promotes muscle & bone healing. As such, it is possible to equate a high protein and acid-forming diet with improved, not bad, bone energy. Although data is conflicting, most studies struggle to explain the theory that the bones are damaged by acid-forming diets. It also suggests that protein, an acidic product, is advantageous.

3.2 pH Grade of the body

When the alkaline diet is taken into account, pH is essential to note.

To put it plainly, pH is a measure on whether something is acidic or alkaline.

The pH values from 0 to 14:

- Alkaline or Basic: 7.1 to 14.0
- Acidic: 0.0 to 6.9
- Neutral value: 7.0

Several advocates of this diet recommend that people track their urine pH to ensure that it is alkaline (< 7) yet not acidic (> 7). It is crucial to remember that the pH within the body varies dramatically. Although some sections are acidic, some alkaline, there is no stated norm. Your stomach is charged with hydrochloric acid, rendering it strongly acidic at a pH of 2-3.5. This

114

acidity is essential for digesting food. In the other side, human blood, with a pH of 7.36–7.44, is often mildly alkaline. It can be lethal if blood pH slips out of the usual range if left unregulated. This only happens under disease circumstances, such as ketoacidosis caused by diabetes, starvation, or alcohol consumption.

The pH-value tests the acidity or alkalinity of a substance. Stomach acid is strongly acidic, to begin with, while blood is mildly alkaline. Food does affect the pH of your urine, but not your semen. It is important that your blood pH remains stable for your wellness.

If you fall beyond the usual range, the cells will fail to live and you will die very soon if not treated. Your body has several successful forms of tightly controlling its pH balance for this purpose. This is considered homeostasis of the acid-base. In reality, adjusting the pH value of blood in healthy individuals is almost unlikely for food, while small variations can exist within the usual range.

Food will modify your urine's pH value, but the result is very uncertain.

The excretion of acids in the pee is one of the key reasons the body monitors the pH in your tissue. A couple of hours later, after you consume a big meal, the urine becomes more acidic, as the body eliminates metabolic waste from the bloodstream. Urine pH is also a weak predictor of total pH in the body and overall well-being. Some factors other than diet may also influence it. The body strongly regulates quantities of blood pH. Diet does not have a major effect on blood pH in healthy people, although it affects the pH in the pee.

3.3 Cancer and Acidity

Many people believe that in an acidic atmosphere cancer only exists and can be cured with an alkaline diet. However, a thorough analysis of the link between diet-mediated acidosis or elevated diet-induced blood acidity and cancer has shown that there is no clear connection. Second, a diet does not affect the pH of the blood substantially. Second, cancer cells are not limited to acidic conditions, even though you believe that food could substantially modify the pH content of blood and other tissues. In fact, cancer spreads across normal, slightly alkaline body tissue (pH 7.4). Several experiments in an alkaline atmosphere have successfully generated cancer cells, and although tumors develop quicker in acidic conditions, tumors themselves generate acidity. Cancer cells do not grow in the acidic environment, but the acidic ecosystem induces cancer cells. There's actually no link between cancer and acid-forming diets. Often, they cultivate cancer cells in alkaline conditions.

3.4 What's a load of acid?

Hundreds of various origins of all-natural ingredients were eaten by our Stone Age ancestors. Game animals & fish were introduced to grains, seeds, veggies, fruits, & roots, providing a pH-balanced diet on avg. In reaction to diets, our organs & body systems have morphed. You should eat acid-forming beans, meat, as well as other enriched protein ingredients, as Nature says, but you have to supplement these with the surplus of alkaline-forming grains, bananas, nuts, spices, and seeds. "You should consume acid-forming beans, meat, as well as other supplemented protein food items, but you have to substitute these with the abundance of alkaline-forming grains, bananas, nuts, spices, and seeds."

3.5 Acidity and Ancestral Diets

From both an ecological as well as a theoretical point of view, examining the acid-alkaline hypothesis reveals disparities. One study reported that 87 percent of early farmers consumed alkaline diets, and the general concept behind the present alkaline diet was constructed. A more recent study reports that, while the other half acid-fed innovation, half of the early farm workers ate alkaline-growing net diets. Notice that our forebears existed in radically distinct ecosystems with linkages to multiple foods. Indeed, acid-forming diets became more popular as individuals drifted away from the southern hemisphere & north (the equator).

Although about half of the poachers had a net diet (acid-forming), it is assumed that modern diseases are much less common (30). Roughly 1/2 of the genetic diets were acidic, particularly among people living outside the equator, according to current studies. Are your foods producing alkaline acids or generating them?

Eating 'alkaline' involves attempting to maintain the body's acid-base pH from 6.5 (slightly acidic) to 7.5. (Alkaline slightly). Our pH can vary in any of the food that we consume. Some foods leave (acidic) by-products in the body when metabolized; others leave alkaline items.

Acid-forming crops include the majority of high materials, such as meat, seafood, eggs & legumes (peas, except alkaline-forming lentils). Everything here is acid-forming starch, caffeine, liquor, & certain crops.

Nearly all fruits & veggies, certain seeds, and nuts, as well as spices, include alkaline-forming meals.

3.6 "Acidic" Food Symbol

- Acid reflux or heartburn

- Fatigue, feeling of being "run down."

- Weight increase

- loss of muscle/Muscle weakness

- Poor ingestion, colonic cramping, tetchy bowel.

- Problems of Urinary tract

- Generic cramps and pains, predominantly in the joints & bones

- Ebbing gums

- Bone harm

- Kidney stones

- Skin glitches

3.7 Common alkaline diet myths

Myth no. 1: From the texture, the acid/alkaline-forming origin of a substance can be determined.

There is no correlation between good flavor and a meal's acid-forming nature. The key factor in pH control is not how the food tastes, but its effect after the body consumes it. A diet is alkalizing because, instead of adding free H_2 to the acid environment, it essentially adds to the bicarbonate (alkalizing compound) atmosphere.

For example, citrus fruits flavor more acidic due to citric acid content, but citric acid is transformed into bicarbonate & water until metabolized. Limes & lemons are often alkalizing, along with the prospect that they taste acidic. In advisement, cranberries & rhubarb (with oxalic acid) often flavor acidic. After metabolization, they remain acidic because both the oxalic acidifier are broken down.

Myth no. 2: For the whole day, the urine pH does not shift.

Although the pH of the blood may remain stable throughout a small range of 7.35 to 7.45 throughout life, the same is not the case with the other pH of fluids, such as saliva and urine, although these may vary during the day. Depending on the food we eat, exercise, depression, and other influences, the pH of the urine increases and decreases. The primary organ is the kidney responsible for the release and

The most accurate calculation is for the first-morning pee after sleeping six hours if you are interested in measuring acid load with a urine pH test. If you can't get up to pee for six hours, weigh the pee in the morning whenever you go for the day, then when you go to pee at night, don't eat or work.

Myth no. 3: Diets do not influence the equilibrium of structural pH.

It is true because during daily metabolic processes the body absorbs a large volume of acid. A large number of acids including those we produce are naturally eliminated, buffered, & excreted. With the strong output of body acid, we will not sustain life. "Considering the critical efficiency of the body to buffer acids it provides, doctors sometimes indicate along the lines of "Don't worry about it

This is true on a larger scale: major changes in pH are serious problems that can be devastating. But it is not important for us to make even significant adjustments. The fact that a small amount of acid deposition may arise from nutritional impairment is something that one's doctor disregards. Acid is called "metabolic acid," as it arises from the digestion of the body, and food in particular.

Myth no. 4: Beef, fish, & seafood producing acids are therefore not healthy for you.

Whether it is from meat, fish, turkey, or any other animal product, or even from beans, these proteins are acid-forming. However, protein intake is essential for human life. The average dietary intake of protein in the USA for adult women is 46 g per day and 56 g per day for males (adults). In fact, when consumed in higher amounts than around 50-60 grams, protein only forms an acid

Usually, if you eat a diet that exceeds 60 g of protein per day, allow ample alkalizing foods to satisfy this extra acid load. To calculate the acid load, track the pH of your first-morning urine and change the intake of alkalizing mineral supplements or alkalizing foods as needed.

Myth No. 5: It is necessary to stop all acid-forming food.

Alkaline diet production would not mean that the diet of all acid-forming products would be zero. A major problem is an equilibrium. Alkaline-forming products and acid-forming products are required for healthy health. Although there may be little need for such acid-forming foods, such as cooked grains or refined sugars, we need adequate nutrition and any protein, whether from animals or plants,

In an alkaline diet, control is the most important aspect. A diet of 65 percent (by mass) alkaline-forming diets and 35 percent acid-forming diets works well in healthy people. For example, if you were to eat a steak (8-ounce) for dinner to retain the 65-35 ratio, you would need to ingest alkaline-forming content (23 ounces) during the day. A ratio of 80-20 of the alkaline content

3.8 How to use the pH document to quantify the acid load

With an easy first-morning urine pH test, you can quantify the metabolic acid load. Note that you just check what we suggest is the urine on the 1st morning before starting your pH testing. We suggest that no additional urine samples or saliva should be evaluated. 'Equilibrated pH' urine is what we are looking for after a night of sleep. When you get up to pee at night, that's fine. You should still quantify the urine in the first hour, as you wake up & sit down. So, be cautious not to feed oneself or get busy once you get up at night to pee. While it is suggested that the pee is checked after 6 hours of continuous sleep, for some people this is not possible, but don't worry. As you wake up, weigh only the first pH of the urine early in the morning.

Get an Alkaline mechanism for the Life pH paper pH Hydrion that calculates the pH ranges from 5.5-8. Tear the 2" of the paper strip and plunge it into a urine sample quickly in the morning (or the pee flow is quickly revealed to the paper strip). Place this moist strip on the tissue to soak excess pee and read it using the defined color code immediately. For first-morning urine, we are looking for the optimal pH variance 6.5-7.5. Below 6.5 implies that the metabolic acids provide an undesirable amount, and satisfactory is every reading around 6.5 & 7.5. The objective is not getting a higher value, simply to be within that limit.

3.9 Wellness Benefits

There is no empirical justification to date for accusations that the alkaline diet would encourage weight loss. Some reports, however, have advised us that the diet could provide some medical welfares.

Diabetes

There is some observational proof on how an alkaline diet can support diabetes tolerance.

66,485 individuals over 14 years were tracked in a 2014 research published in the German newspaper Diabetologia. There have been 1,372 recent diabetes conclusions at this point. 7 Tests have shown that those with more acid-forming foods have a slightly augmented chance of evolving diabetes through their testing.

The writers of the study say that large feasting of acid-forming foods can be due to insulin resistance, a condition directly allied to diabetes.

Masses of muscles

As you develop and have an important component to avoid bone breaks and falls, it will help you maintain muscle mass while following an alkaline diet.

A three-year clinical study of 384 women and men (aged 65 and above) reported in the American Journal of Clinical Nutrition in 2008 showed that high intakes of potassium-rich foods, such as vegetables and fruits recommended as the basis for an alkaline diet, can help older adults retain muscle mass as they mature.

Researcher's scrutinized data on 2,689 individuals aged 18 and 79 years in another 2013 research conducted in Osteoporosis International. They developed a "limited yet important" correlation between alkaline diet adherence and mass muscle preservation.

Cardiac Disorder

Higher mortality rates could be linked with a high acid discharge diet, but the data is conflicting. Researchers find that individuals with the highest PRAL have seen a substantial increase in coronary atherosclerotic disease in a 2016 analysis published in Cardiovascular Diabetology, and appear to belong to the high-risk category relative to those with the lowest PRAL ratings.

A second study, though, showed that both extremely acidic and intensely alkaline diets had higher death rates, while for those on a more usual diet, life was longer.

The study analyzed findings from the Swedish Mammography Survey and the Swedish Male Survey reported in the Journal of Diet, which involved 36,740 persons out of 44,957 males over a 15-year follow-up duration. Researchers observed higher mortality rates in both men and women in people with a heavy nutritional or alkaline load intake, in comparison to those with a healthy diet with an acid foundation.

Chronic Kidney Disorder (CKD)

Rising dietary acid content is said to recover metabolic acidosis and increase the likelihood of contracting kidney disease.

In a study published in the 2015 American Journal of Nephrology, researchers tracked 15,055 people without kidney disease across 21 years (who were a fragment of the Atherosclerosis Prevention Research in Societies) and noted that a higher dietary acid load was associated with a higher risk of chronic kidney disorder after correction for other variables (such as genetic factors, calorie intake, and demographics)

The greater consumption of magnesium and vegetable protein items are the most important protective correlation of kidney disease with separate dietary ingredients.

Danger of Fracture

It is suspected that a heavily acidic diet improves the likelihood of fractures and osteoporosis in older adults. The hypothesis is that to reduce acidity, the body leeches calcium, an alkaline material, from the bones.

3.10 The Last Say

Alkaline diets appear to have a pH that is more alkaline in the urine, which may contribute to less calcium in the urine. However, this does not represent the overall calcium content owing to some buffers, including phosphate, as seen in some recent lessons. No substantial proof exists that this reinforces the defense of the bone or protects against osteoporosis. Alkaline diets, however, can result in a variety of health benefits, as described below.

1. The K/Na ratio would be increased by increased vegetables and fruit alkaline diet and could promote bone strength, decrease muscle wastage, and decrease other chronic diseases such as hypertension and strokes.

2. Many benefits from physical well-being to performance and learning by the subsequent increase of growth hormone may be improved by an alkaline diet.

3. Another added advantage of the alkaline diet is the growth of intracellular magnesium, which is important for many enzyme systems. In the vitamin D apocrine/exocrine systems, accessible magnesium, which is required to enable vitamin D, can contribute to several added benefits.

4. For those chemotherapeutic agents which need a higher pH, alkalinity can result in additional benefits.

It is advisable to recommend an alkaline diet from the analysis mentioned above to reduce the mortality and morbidity of chronic diseases that influence our elderly population. One of the first factors of an alkaline diet that contains more vegetables and berries is understanding what kind of soil they have been made, as the mineral content can be strongly influenced by this. There is a little scientific study in this field at this stage, but some further studies on muscle influence, growth hormone, while vitamin D interaction is expected.

Conclusion

It is necessary to maintain a balance in your life, regardless of what path you take. Since acidic components rule our lifestyle, it has become more important to have an alkaline diet. The widespread use of chemical medicines has further affected the immune systems of everyday citizens, making them susceptible to the complex diseases of today's planet. Dr. Sebi struggled against this lifestyle, and he enjoyed some serious breakthroughs in his career that were well demonstrated in the previous chapters. If we turn from our western way of life to the acts of nature, we will remove some illnesses and cure others. Dr. Alfredo Bowman's thesis was supported by recent findings and experiments in the field of herbal medicine. The herbal ingredients that makeup Dr. Sebi's diet plan are all the carbohydrates and vitamins important to our body. In the fight against diseases which, unlike the chemical treatments of the same topic, are considered severe and sometimes untreatable in the medical sciences today with minimum side effects, his medicines have also shown substantial results.

CPSIA information can be obtained
at www.ICGtesting.com
Printed in the USA
BVHW061001130421
604816BV00005B/1150